IMPROVING CHILD NUTRITION

The achievable imperative
for global progress

CONTENTS

FOREWORD

Poor nutrition in the first 1,000 days of children's lives can have irreversible consequences. For millions of children, it means they are, forever, stunted.

Smaller than their non-stunted peers, stunted children are more susceptible to sickness. In school, they often fall behind in class. They enter adulthood more likely to become overweight and more prone to non-communicable disease. And when they start work, they often earn less than their non-stunted co-workers.

It is difficult to think of a greater injustice than robbing a child, in the womb and in infancy, of the ability to fully develop his or her talents throughout life.

This is a tragedy for the 165 million children under the age of 5 afflicted by stunting in the world today. It is a violation of their rights. It is also a huge burden for nations whose future citizens will be neither as healthy nor as productive as they could have been.

And let us not forget the tens of millions of children around the world who are vulnerable to the ravages of life-threatening, severe acute malnutrition. Slowly, treatment is expanding but, still, too many children remain out of its reach. About one third of under-five mortality is attributable to undernutrition.

At last, the gravity of undernutrition and its long-term effects are being acknowledged and acted upon – with increasing urgency. This is, in large part, in recognition of the ever-growing body of compelling evidence on the short- and long-term impacts of stunting and other forms of undernutrition.

Recognizing that investing in nutrition is a key way to advance global welfare, the G8 has put this high on its agenda. The global nutrition community is uniting around the Scaling Up Nutrition movement. The United Nations Secretary-General has included elimination of stunting as a goal in his Zero Hunger Challenge to the world. The 2013 World Economic Forum highlighted food and nutrition security as a global priority. And a panel of top economists from the most recent Copenhagen Consensus selected stunting reduction as a top investment priority.

More and more countries are scaling up their nutrition programmes to reach children during the critical period from pregnancy to the age of 2. These programmes are working. Countries that are reaching mothers and children with effective nutrition and related interventions during the first 1,000 days are achieving results. Stunting and other forms of undernutrition are decreasing.

But we must still reach millions of mothers and their children, especially those in the hardest to reach areas. Urgently.

The World Health Assembly has set the goal of achieving a 40 per cent reduction in the number of stunted children under 5 years old by 2025, or around 70 million children saved from the misery of stunting.

This report shows that we can attain that target. Countries like Ethiopia, Haiti, Nepal, Peru and Rwanda are leading the way, quickly scaling up equity-focused initiatives. Committed to results, they are achieving progress through advocacy, better allocation of resources and investments in tailored policies and programmes.

And where progress can be made, we have a moral obligation to do so.

The legacy of the first 1,000 days of a child's life can last forever. So, we must do what we can, as fast as we can, to give the most disadvantaged mothers and children dependable, quality nutrition.

The right start in life is a healthy start – and that is the only start from which children can realize their promise and potential. We owe that to every child, everywhere.

Anthony Lake
Executive Director, UNICEF

KEY MESSAGES

Focus on stunting prevention

- Globally, about one in four children under 5 years old are stunted (26 per cent in 2011). An estimated 80 per cent of the world's 165 million stunted children live in just 14 countries.

- Stunting and other forms of undernutrition reduce a child's chance of survival, while also hindering optimal health and growth. Stunting is associated with suboptimal brain development, which is likely to have long-lasting harmful consequences for cognitive ability, school performance and future earnings. This in turn affects the development potential of nations.

- In tackling child undernutrition, there has been a shift from efforts to reduce underweight prevalence (inadequate weight for age) to prevention of stunting (inadequate length/height for age). There is better understanding of the crucial importance of nutrition during the critical 1,000-day period covering pregnancy and the first two years of the child's life, and of the fact that stunting reflects deficiencies during this period. The World Health Assembly has adopted a new target of reducing the number of stunted children under the age of 5 by 40 per cent by 2025.

- In addition to the quality and frequency of infant and young child feeding and the incidence of infectious diseases, the mother's nutrition and health status are important determinants of stunting. An undernourished mother is more likely to give birth to a stunted child, perpetuating a vicious cycle of undernutrition and poverty.

- A stunted child enters adulthood with a greater propensity for developing obesity and chronic diseases. With increasing urbanization and shifts in diet and lifestyle, the result could be a burgeoning epidemic of such conditions in many low- and middle-income countries. This would create new economic and social challenges, especially among vulnerable groups.

Approaches that work

- Reductions in stunting and other forms of undernutrition can be achieved through proven interventions. These include improving women's nutrition, especially before, during and after pregnancy; early and exclusive breastfeeding; timely, safe, appropriate and high-quality complementary food; and appropriate micronutrient interventions.

- Timing is important – interventions should focus on the critical 1,000-day window including pregnancy and before a child turns 2. After that window closes, disproportionate weight gain may increase the child's risk of becoming overweight and developing other health problems.

- Efforts to scale up nutrition programmes are working, benefiting women and children and their communities in many countries. Such programmes all have common elements: political commitment, national policies and programmes based on sound evidence and analysis, the presence of trained and skilled community workers collaborating with communities, effective communication and advocacy, and multi-sectoral, integrated service delivery.

Global momentum to scale up nutrition

- Globally, interest in nutrition has increased dramatically. Recurrent food shortages, rising food prices, strengthened evidence and rising obesity have created the impetus for widespread concern and action.

- More than ever, investing in nutrition is seen as a key development priority to benefit global welfare. The Group of 8 (G8) of the world's wealthiest countries has put nutrition high on its development agenda, and the United Nations Secretary-General's Zero Hunger Challenge includes the elimination of stunting as a goal.

- The global nutrition community is uniting around the Scaling Up Nutrition (SUN) movement, which supports nationally driven processes for the reduction of stunting and other forms of malnutrition.

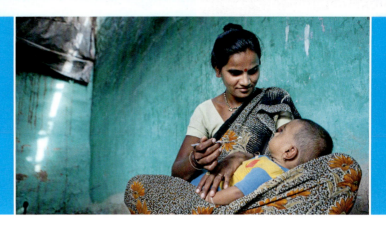

Chapter 1

INTRODUCTION

UNICEF's 2009 report *Tracking Progress on Child and Maternal Nutrition* drew attention to the impact of high levels of undernutrition on child survival, growth and development and their social and economic toll on nations. It described the state of nutrition programmes worldwide and argued for improving and expanding delivery of key nutrition interventions during the critical 1,000-day window covering a woman's pregnancy and the first two years of her child's life, when rapid physical and mental development occurs. This report builds on those earlier findings by highlighting new developments and demonstrating that efforts to scale up nutrition programmes are working, benefiting children in many countries.

UNICEF first outlined the nature and determinants of maternal and child undernutrition in a conceptual framework more than two decades ago. Child undernutrition is caused not just by the lack of adequate, nutritious food, but by frequent illness, poor care practices and lack of access to health and other social services. This conceptual framework is as relevant today as it was then, but it is now influenced by recent shifts and exciting developments in the field of nutrition.

Strengthened by new evidence, an understanding of the short- and long-term consequences of undernutrition has evolved. There is even stronger confirmation that undernutrition can trap children, families, communities and nations in an intergenerational cycle of poor nutrition, illness and poverty. More is known about the mechanisms that link inadequate growth due to nutritional deficiencies before the age of 2 with impaired brain development and subsequent reduced performance in school. And there is clearer, more comprehensive evidence of the need to promote optimal growth during this critical period

to avoid an elevated risk of non-communicable diseases, such as cardiovascular disease, in adulthood and even in the next generation.

Equipped with this new knowledge, the international community now places more emphasis on stunting (inadequate length/height for age) as the indicator of choice for measuring progress towards reducing undernutrition. This means focusing less on underweight (inadequate weight for age), which is a key indicator for measuring progress towards Millennium Development Goal (MDG) 1.

In May 2012, the World Health Assembly, the decision-making body of the World Health Organization (WHO), agreed on a new target: reducing the number of stunted children under the age of 5 by 40 per cent by 2025. The United Nations Secretary-General has included elimination of stunting as a goal in his Zero Hunger Challenge, launched in June 2012. This emphasis on stunting has led to a review of national programmes and strategies to increase the focus on prevention and integrated programmes.

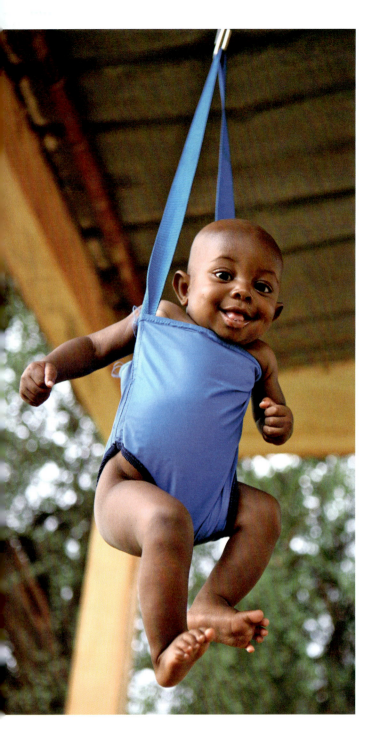

In addition to the shift in emphasis towards reducing stunting, there has been a major shift in the global nutrition landscape, sparking unprecedented momentum for action. Just a few years ago, nutrition was a neglected area of development, and the nutrition community was fragmented, lacking a common voice or unified approach. The initiation of the SUN movement in 2010 brought about much-needed change.

The SUN movement seeks to build national commitment to accelerate progress to reduce stunting and other forms of undernutrition, as well as overweight. Through SUN, countries are working to increase access to affordable and nutritious food, as well as demand for it. They are also addressing the other factors that determine nutritional status, such as improved feeding and care practices, clean water, sanitation, health care, social protection and initiatives to empower women.

More than 30 countries in Africa, Asia and Latin America have joined SUN. They are expanding their nutrition programmes, supported by donor countries, United Nations organizations, civil society and the private sector. SUN is assisting nations in meeting their obligations to ensure fulfilment of their citizens' right to food. As initially codified in the Universal Declaration of Human Rights and reaffirmed by the International Covenant on Economic, Social and Cultural Rights, the right to food is a fundamental human right. Realizing the right to food is critical to fulfilling other rights, most importantly the right to health and the opportunities that it conveys.

Stunting and other forms of undernutrition epitomize societal inequities, and stunting serves as a marker for poverty and underdevelopment. This report shows that there is now an opportunity to address this major inequity by scaling up nutrition programming.

To show that results can be achieved, even within a short time frame, the report includes case studies from countries where nutrition has been improved at scale. It also presents an updated picture of the status of nutrition and profiles countries where the prevalence of stunting in children under the age of 5 is 40 per cent or higher, as well as those with the highest absolute burden of stunting.

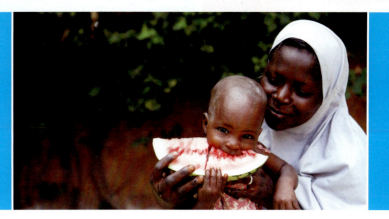

Chapter 2

CAUSES AND CONSEQUENCES OF UNDERNUTRITION

Causes and timing of undernutrition

The UNICEF conceptual framework defines nutrition and captures the multifactorial causality of undernutrition *(Figure 1)*. Nutritional status is influenced by three broad factors: food, health and care. Optimal nutritional status results when children have access to affordable, diverse, nutrient-rich food; appropriate maternal and child-care practices; adequate health services; and a healthy environment including safe water, sanitation and good hygiene practices. These factors directly influence nutrient intake and the presence of disease. The interaction between undernutrition and infection creates a potentially lethal cycle of worsening illness and deteriorating nutritional status.

Food, health and care are affected by social, economic and political factors. The combination and relative importance of these factors differ from country to country. Understanding the immediate and underlying causes of undernutrition in a given context is critical to delivering appropriate, effective and sustainable solutions and adequately meeting the needs of the most vulnerable people.

From a life-cycle perspective, the most crucial time to meet a child's nutritional requirements is in the 1,000 days including the period of pregnancy and ending with the child's second birthday. During this time, the child has increased nutritional needs to support rapid growth and development, is more susceptible to infections, has heightened sensitivity to biological programming[1] and is totally dependent on others for nutrition, care and social interactions.

Child undernutrition is assessed by measuring height and weight and screening for clinical manifestations and biochemical markers. Indicators based on weight, height and age are compared to international standards and are most commonly used to assess the nutritional status of a population. Stunting (inadequate length/height for age) captures early chronic exposure to undernutrition; wasting (inadequate weight for height) captures acute undernutrition; underweight (inadequate weight for age) is a composite indicator that includes elements of stunting and wasting.

Today's concerted focus on reducing stunting reflects an improved understanding of the importance of undernutrition during the most critical period of development in early life and of the long-term consequences extending into adulthood. Evidence from 54 low- and middle-income countries indicates that growth faltering on average begins during pregnancy and continues to about 24 months of age. This loss in linear growth is not recovered, and catch-up growth later on in childhood is minimal.[2] While the UNICEF conceptual framework reflected a focus on children of preschool age, there is now more emphasis on policies and programmes that support action before the age of 2 years, especially on maternal nutrition and health and appropriate infant and young child feeding and care practices.

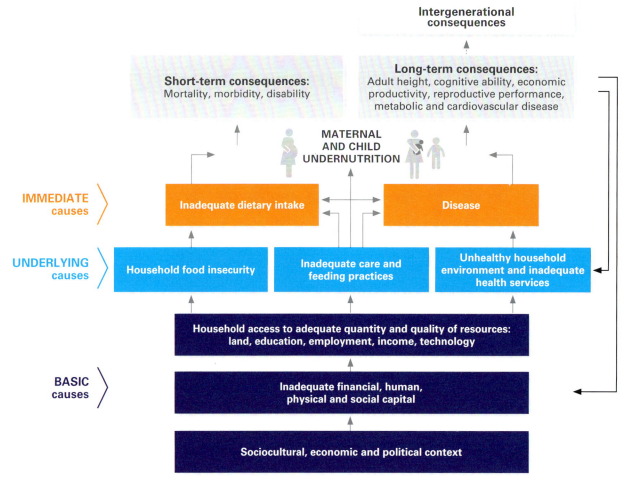

The black arrows show that the consequences of undernutrition can feed back to the underlying and basic causes of undernutrition, perpetuating the cycle of undernutrition, poverty and inequities.

Source: Adapted from UNICEF, 1990.

Adequate maternal nutrition, health and physical status are crucial to prevent child undernutrition. Pregnancy increases nutrient needs, and protein, energy, vitamin and mineral deficiencies are common during pregnancy. Deficiencies are not solely the result of inadequate dietary intake: Disease can impair absorption of nutrients and reduce appetite, and environmental and psychosocial stress affecting the mother can contribute to child undernutrition.[3] Poor maternal nutrition impairs foetal development and contributes to low birthweight, subsequent stunting and other forms of undernutrition.

Undernourished girls have a greater likelihood of becoming undernourished mothers who in turn have a greater chance of giving birth to low birthweight babies,[4] perpetuating an intergenerational cycle. This cycle can be compounded further in young mothers, especially adolescent girls who begin childbearing before attaining adequate growth and development. Short intervals between pregnancies and having several children may accumulate or exacerbate nutrition deficits, passing these deficiencies on to the children.

Low birthweight is associated with increased morbidity and mortality: An estimated 60 to 80 per cent of neonatal deaths occur among low birthweight babies (2005 estimate).[5] In South Asia, an estimated 28 per cent of infants are born with low birthweight.[6]

After birth, a number of practices can directly lead to poor growth: inadequate breastfeeding practices such as non-exclusive breastfeeding; inappropriate complementary feeding, such as starting at the wrong age; poor access to or use of diverse types of food and inadequate intake of micronutrients. Poor growth can be aggravated further by frequent incidence of infectious diseases like diarrhoea, malaria or infestation with intestinal worms.

Consequences of undernutrition

Stunting and other forms of undernutrition are clearly a major contributing factor to child mortality, disease and disability. For example, a severely stunted child faces a four times higher risk of dying, and a severely wasted child is at a nine times higher risk.[7] Specific nutritional deficiencies such as vitamin A, iron or zinc deficiency also increase risk of death. Undernutrition can cause various diseases such as blindness due to vitamin A deficiency and neural tube defects due to folic acid deficiency.

The broader understanding of the devastating consequences of undernutrition on morbidity and mortality is based on well-established evidence. Knowledge of the impact of stunting and other forms of undernutrition on social and economic development and human capital formation has been supported and expanded by more recent research.[8]

Earlier research clarified the harmful impact of inadequate intake of specific micronutrients such as iron, folic acid and iodine on development of the brain and nervous system and on subsequent school performance. The impact of iron deficiency, which reduces school performance in children and the physical capacity for work among adults, has also been documented.

Undernutrition early in life clearly has major consequences for future educational, income and productivity outcomes. Stunting is associated with poor school achievement and poor school performance.[9] Recent longitudinal studies among cohorts of children from Brazil, Guatemala, India, the Philippines and South Africa confirmed the association between stunting and a reduction in schooling, and also found that stunting was a predictor of grade failure.[10]

Reduced school attendance and educational outcomes result in diminished income-earning capacity in adulthood. A 2007 study estimated an average 22 per cent loss of yearly income in adulthood.[11]

What is now becoming clearer is that the developmental impact of stunting and other forms of undernutrition happens earlier and is greater than previously thought. Brain and nervous system development begins early in pregnancy and is largely complete by the time the child reaches the age of 2. The timing, severity and duration of nutritional deficiencies during this period affect brain development in different ways, influenced by the brain's need for a given nutrient at a specific time.[12] While the developing brain has the capacity for repair, it is also highly vulnerable, and nutrient deficiencies during critical periods have long-term effects.

This new knowledge, together with the evidence that the irreversible process of stunting happens early in life, has led to a shift in programming focus. Previously the emphasis was on children under age 5, while now it is increasingly on the 1,000-day period up to age 2, including pregnancy.

Improvements in nutrition after age 2 do not usually lead to recovery of lost potential. Data from the five countries studied indicated that weight gain during the first two years of life, but not afterwards, improved school performance later on in childhood, underlining the critical importance of this window of opportunity.[13] Earlier studies of malnourished Korean orphans adopted into American families showed residual poor performance on cognitive tests based on nutritional status at the time of adoption. Adoption before age 2 was associated with significantly higher cognitive test scores compared with children adopted later.[14] A series of longitudinal South African studies assessed the impact of severe undernutrition before age 2 on physical growth and intellectual functioning in adolescence. Even accounting for improvements in environment and catch-up growth, the children who had experienced chronic undernutrition in early infancy suffered from irreversible intellectual impairment.[15]

A consequence that is also emerging more clearly is the impact of stunting and subsequent disproportionate and rapid weight gain on health later in life.

These long-term effects are referred to as the foetal programming concept: Poor foetal growth, small size at birth and continued poor growth in early life followed by rapid weight gain later in childhood raises the risk of coronary heart disease, stroke, hypertension and type II diabetes.[16] Attaining optimal growth before 24 months of age is desirable; becoming stunted but then gaining weight disproportionately after 24 months is likely to increase the risk of becoming overweight and developing other health problems.[17]

As stunted children enter adulthood with a greater propensity for developing obesity and other chronic diseases, the possibility of a burgeoning epidemic of poor health opens up, especially in transitional countries experiencing increasing urbanization and shifts in diet and lifestyle. This epidemiological transition could create new economic and social challenges in many low- and middle-income countries where stunting is prevalent, especially among poorer population groups.

BOX 1   The lethal interaction between undernutrition and common infections

An estimated one third of deaths among children under age 5 are attributed to undernutrition. Undernutrition puts children at far greater risk of death and severe illness due to common childhood infections, such as pneumonia, diarrhoea, malaria, HIV and AIDS and measles. A child who is severely underweight is 9.5 times more likely to die of diarrhoea than a child who is not, and for a stunted child the risk of death is 4.6 times higher *(Figure 2)*.

Undernutrition weakens the immune system, putting children at higher risk of more severe, frequent and prolonged bouts of illness. Undernutrition is also a consequence of repeated infections, which may further worsen the child's nutritional status at a time of greater nutritional needs. This interaction between undernutrition and infection creates a potentially lethal cycle of worsening illness and deteriorating nutritional status.

Critical nutrition interventions that break this cycle include promoting optimal breastfeeding practices, encouraging micronutrient supplementation and reducing the incidence of low birthweight *(see Chapter 4)*. For example, infants not breastfed are 15 times more likely to die from pneumonia and 11 times more likely to die from diarrhoea than children who are exclusively breastfed *(Figure 3)*. Similarly, all-cause mortality is 14 times higher for infants not breastfeeding than for exclusively breastfed children.[18]

FIGURE 2   Undernourished children are at higher risk of death from diarrhoea or pneumonia

Odds ratio of dying from diarrhoea or pneumonia among undernourished children relative to well-nourished children, in selected countries*

	Odds ratio			
	Severe undernutrition	**Moderate undernutrition**	**Mild undernutrition**	**No undernutrition**
Underweight				
Diarrhoea	9.5	3.4	2.1	1.0
Pneumonia	6.4	1.3	1.2	1.0
Stunting				
Diarrhoea	4.6	1.6	1.2	1.0
Pneumonia	3.2	1.3	1.0	1.0
Wasting				
Diarrhoea	6.3	2.9	1.2	1.0
Pneumonia	8.7	4.2	1.6	1.0

* Bangladesh, Ghana, Guinea-Bissau, India, Nepal, Pakistan, the Philippines and Senegal.

Source: Adapted from Black et al., 'Maternal and Child Undernutrition: Global and regional exposures and health consequences', *Lancet*, vol. 371, no. 9608, 19 January 2008, pp. 243–260.

FIGURE 3   Infants who are not breastfed are at a greater risk of death from diarrhoea or pneumonia than infants who are breastfed

Relative risk of diarrhoea and pneumonia incidence and mortality among infants 0–5 months old who are not breastfed, partially breastfed and exclusively breastfed

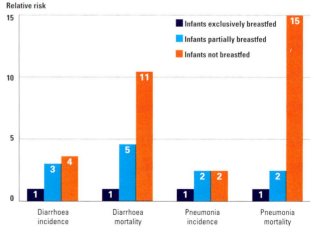

Source: Adapted from Black et al., 'Maternal and Child Undernutrition: Global and regional exposures and health consequences', *Lancet*, vol. 371, no. 9608, 19 January 2008, pp. 243–260.

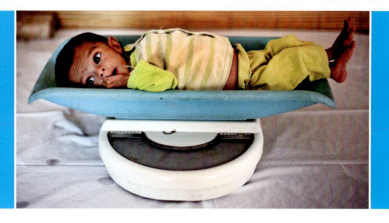

Chapter **3**

CURRENT STATUS OF NUTRITION

Child malnutrition can manifest itself in several ways. It is most commonly assessed through measurement of a child's weight and height, as well as through biochemical and clinical assessment. This chapter reports on the levels and trends of the anthropometric indicators of nutritional status, gathered from data collected through large nationally representative household surveys.[19]

BOX 2 | **Definitions of anthropometric indicators**

- **Stunting** reflects chronic undernutrition during the most critical periods of growth and development in early life. It is defined as the percentage of children aged 0 to 59 months whose height for age is below minus two standard deviations (moderate and severe stunting) and minus three standard deviations (severe stunting) from the median of the WHO Child Growth Standards.

- **Underweight** is a composite form of undernutrition that includes elements of stunting and wasting. It is defined as the percentage of children aged 0 to 59 months whose weight for age is below minus two

standard deviations (moderate and severe underweight) and minus three standard deviations (severe underweight) from the median of the WHO Child Growth Standards.

- **Wasting** reflects acute undernutrition. It is defined as the percentage of children aged 0 to 59 months whose weight for height is below minus two standard deviations (moderate and severe wasting) and minus three standard deviations (severe wasting) from the median of the WHO Child Growth Standards.

- **Severe acute malnutrition** is defined as the percentage of children aged 6 to 59 months whose weight for

height is below minus three standard deviations from the median of the WHO Child Growth Standards, or by a mid-upper-arm circumference less than 115 mm, with or without nutritional oedema.

- **Overweight** is defined as the percentage of children aged 0 to 59 months whose weight for height is above two standard deviations (overweight and obese) or above three standard deviations (obese) from the median of the WHO Child Growth Standards.

- **Low birthweight** is defined as a weight of less than 2,500 grams at birth.

Stunting

Globally, more than one quarter (26 per cent) of children under 5 years of age were stunted in 2011 – roughly 165 million children worldwide.[20] But this burden is not evenly distributed around the world. Sub-Saharan Africa and South Asia are home to three fourths of the world's stunted children *(Figure 4)*. In sub-Saharan Africa, 40 per cent of children under 5 years of age are stunted; in South Asia, 39 per cent are stunted.

Fourteen countries are home to 80 per cent of the world's stunted children *(Figure 5)*. The 24 countries profiled beginning on page 55 of this report include the ten countries with the greatest absolute burden of stunted children, together with countries that have very high stunting prevalence, at 40 per cent or above *(Figure 6)*. All but five of the 24 countries profiled are in sub-Saharan Africa or South Asia. In the four countries with the highest prevalence (Timor-Leste, Burundi, Niger and Madagascar), more than half of children under 5 years old are stunted.

Stunting trends

The global prevalence of stunting in children under the age of 5 has declined 36 per cent over the past two decades – from an estimated 40 per cent in 1990 to 26 per cent in 2011. This is an average annual rate of reduction of 2.1 per cent per year. In fact, every region has observed reductions in stunting prevalence over the past two decades *(Figure 7)*, and some regions have achieved remarkable improvements.

The greatest declines in stunting prevalence occurred in East Asia and the Pacific. This region experienced about a 70 per cent reduction in prevalence – from 42 per cent in 1990 to 12 per cent in 2011. This major reduction was largely due to improvements made by China. The prevalence of stunting in China decreased from more than 30 per cent in 1990 to 10 per cent in 2010.

Latin America and the Caribbean reduced stunting prevalence by nearly half during this same period. The South Asia and Middle East and North Africa regions have both achieved more than a one-third reduction in stunting prevalence since 1990.

FIGURE 4   **Stunting prevalence is highest in sub-Saharan Africa and South Asia**

Percentage of children under age 5 who are moderately or severely stunted

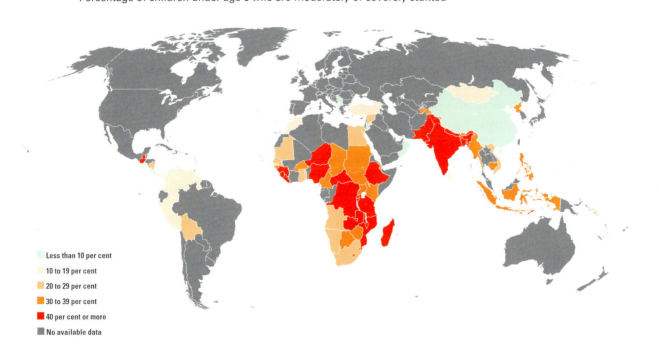

- Less than 10 per cent
- 10 to 19 per cent
- 20 to 29 per cent
- 30 to 39 per cent
- 40 per cent or more
- No available data

Note: Data are from 2007 to 2011, except for India.

This map is stylized and not to scale. It does not reflect a position by UNICEF on the legal status of any country or territory or the delimitation of any frontiers. The dotted line between Jammu and Kashmir represents approximately the Line of Control agreed upon by India and Pakistan. The final status of Jammu and Kashmir has not yet been agreed upon by the Parties. The final boundary between the Republic of the Sudan and the Republic of South Sudan has not yet been determined.

Source: UNICEF Global Nutrition Database, 2012, based on Multiple Indicator Cluster Surveys (MICS), Demographic and Health Surveys (DHS) and other national surveys.

FIGURE 5

FIGURE 5 — 80 per cent of the world's stunted children live in 14 countries

14 countries with the largest numbers of children under 5 years old who are moderately or severely stunted

Ranking	Country	Year	Stunting prevalence (%)	% of global burden (2011)	Number of stunted children (moderate or severe, thousands)
1	**India**	2005–2006	48	38	61,723
2	**Nigeria**	2008	41	7	11,049
3	**Pakistan**	2011	44	6	9,663
4	**China**	2010	10	5	8,059
5	**Indonesia**	2010	36	5	7,547
6	**Bangladesh**	2011	41	4	5,958
7	**Ethiopia**	2011	44	3	5,291
8	**Democratic Republic of the Congo**	2010	43	3	5,228
9	**Philippines**	2008	32	2	3,602
10	**United Republic of Tanzania**	2010	42	2	3,475
11	Egypt	2008	29	2	2,628
12	Kenya	2008–2009	35	1	2,403
13	Uganda	2011	33	1	2,219
14	Sudan	2010	35	1	1,744

Note: The countries in bold are profiled beginning on page 55 of this report. Updated data from Afghanistan and Yemen were not available, but these countries are likely to contribute significantly to the global burden of stunting – last reported data of stunting prevalence were 59 per cent for Afghanistan in 2004 and 58 per cent for Yemen in 2003.

Source: UNICEF Global Nutrition Database, 2012, based on MICS, DHS and other national surveys, 2007–2011, except for India.

FIGURE 6 — 21 countries have very high stunting prevalence

Percentage of children under age 5 who are moderately or severely stunted, in 21 countries where prevalence is at least 40 per cent

Country	Year	Stunting prevalence (%)
Timor-Leste	2009–2010	58
Burundi	2010	58
Niger	2011	51
Madagascar	2008–2009	50
India	2005–2006	48
Guatemala	2008–2009	48
Malawi	2010	47
Zambia	2007	45
Ethiopia	2011	44
Sierra Leone	2010	44
Rwanda	2010	44
Pakistan	2011	44
Democratic Republic of the Congo	2010	43
Mozambique	2011	43
United Republic of Tanzania	2010	42
Liberia	2010	42
Bangladesh	2011	41
Central African Republic	2010	41
Nigeria	2008	41
Nepal	2011	41
Guinea	2008	40

Note: The countries in bold are profiled beginning on page 55 of this report.

Source: UNICEF Global Nutrition Database, 2012, based on MICS, DHS and other national surveys, 2007–2011, except for India.

FIGURE 7 — All regions have reduced stunting prevalence since 1990

Percentage of children under age 5 who are moderately or severely stunted and percentage reduction, 1990–2011

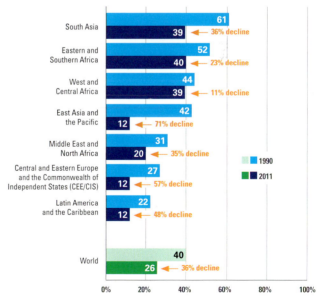

Source: UNICEF, WHO, World Bank, *Joint Child Malnutrition Estimates*, 2012.

However, progress in reducing stunting prevalence in sub-Saharan Africa was limited to 16 per cent, from 47 per cent in 1990 to 40 per cent in 2011. More than one third of countries in sub-Saharan Africa have very high stunting prevalence.

Disparities in stunting

Regional and national averages can hide important disparities among subnational population groups – such as by gender, household wealth and area of residence. Globally, over one third of children in rural households are stunted compared to one quarter in urban households *(Figure 8)*. Children in the poorest households are more than twice as likely to be stunted as children in the richest households. In the regions with the highest rates of stunting – sub-Saharan Africa and South Asia – the proportion of stunted children under 5 in the poorest households compared with the proportion in the richest households ranges from nearly twice as high in sub-Saharan Africa (48 per cent versus 25 per cent) to more than twice as high in South Asia (59 per cent versus 25 per cent).

Girls and boys are almost equally likely to be stunted globally, but in sub-Saharan Africa stunting afflicts more boys (42 per cent) than girls (36 per cent) *(Figure 9)*.

FIGURE 8 **The poorest children and those living in rural areas are those more often stunted**

Percentage of children under age 5 who are moderately or severely stunted, by selected background characteristics

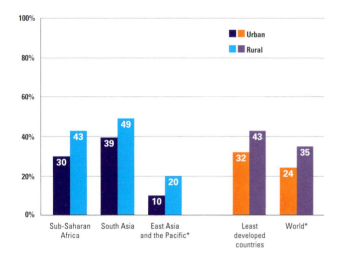

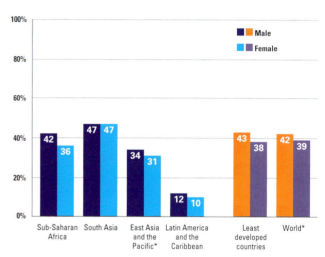

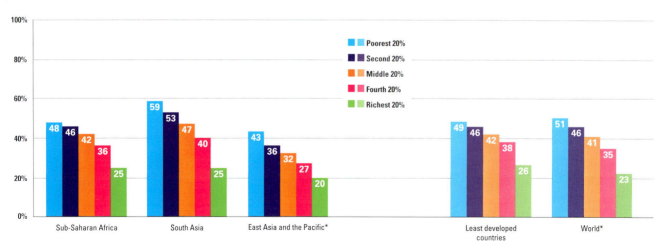

* Excludes China.

Note: Analysis is based on a subset of countries with available data by subnational groupings and regional estimates are presented only where adequate coverage is met. Data from 2007 to 2011, except for Brazil and India.

Source: UNICEF Global Nutrition Database, 2012, based on MICS, DHS and other national surveys.

FIGURE 9 In sub-Saharan Africa, stunting is more prevalent in boys than in girls

Ratio of moderate or severe stunting prevalence (girls to boys) among children 0–59 months, in sub-Saharan countries with available data

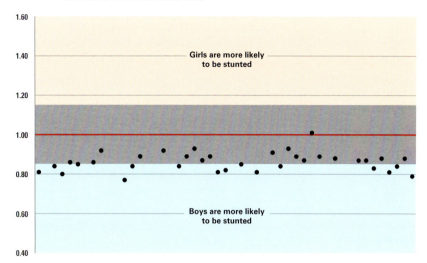

How to read this graph:
For the purpose of illustrating gender equity, a range from 0.85 to 1.15 in the ratio of stunting prevalence was taken as the window of 'gender parity' (grey band). A dot above the grey band would suggest that girls are more likely to be stunted, while a dot below the band suggests that boys are more likely to be stunted.

Source: UNICEF Global Nutrition Database, 2012, based on MICS, DHS and other national surveys, 2007–2011.

BOX 3 The double burden of malnutrition

The coexistence of stunting and overweight, or the double burden of malnutrition, presents a unique programmatic challenge in countries where relatively high rates of both stunting and overweight persist among the country's under-five population. Global trends in the prevalence of stunting and overweight among children under age 5 have moved in opposite directions since 1990 *(Figure 10)*. Compared to two decades ago, today there are 54 per cent more overweight children globally and 35 per cent fewer stunted children. For example, in Indonesia, one in three children under age 5 are moderately or severely stunted (36 per cent) while at the same time one in seven is overweight (14 per cent). Efforts are needed in 'double burden' countries to promote good infant and young child feeding practices that support linear growth without causing excessive weight gain.

FIGURE 10 Contrasting global trends in child stunting and overweight

Percentage and number of children under age 5 who are moderately or severely stunted and who are overweight

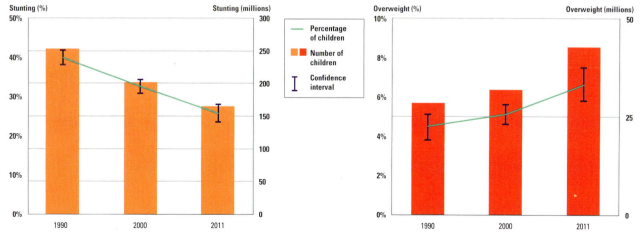

Note: The lines (with 95 per cent confidence intervals) reflect the percentages of children and the bars reflect the numbers of children.

Source: UNICEF, WHO, World Bank, *Joint Child Malnutrition Estimates*, 2012.

Underweight

Globally in 2011, an estimated 101 million children under 5 years of age were underweight, or approximately 16 per cent of children under 5. Underweight prevalence is highest in South Asia, which has a rate of 33 per cent, followed by sub-Saharan Africa, at 21 per cent. South Asia has 59 million underweight children, while sub-Saharan Africa has 30 million.

The prevalence of underweight children under age 5 is an indicator to measure progress towards MDG 1, which aims to halve the proportion of people who suffer from hunger between 1990 and 2015. Globally, underweight prevalence has declined, from 25 per cent in 1990 to 16 per cent today – a 37 per cent reduction. The greatest reductions have been achieved in Central and Eastern Europe and the Commonwealth of Independent States, where prevalence has declined by 87 per cent, and in East Asia and the Pacific, where it fell 73 per cent (as with stunting, driven largely in the latter region by reductions made in China). In other regions, progress remained slow; in sub-Saharan Africa underweight prevalence dropped by 26 per cent.

As of 2011, 30 countries were on track to meet the MDG 1 target, 25 countries had made insufficient progress and 12 countries had made no progress *(Figure 11)*. Of the 24 countries profiled in this report, only 8 are on track to achieve the MDG 1 target. While countries make progress towards the target by decreasing underweight prevalence, these declines may represent an accompanying transition towards a higher prevalence of overweight with persistent levels of stunting.

FIGURE 11 **MDG 1 progress: 30 countries 'on track' as of 2011**

Country progress towards MDG 1 target to halve, between 1990 and 2015, the proportion of people who suffer from hunger

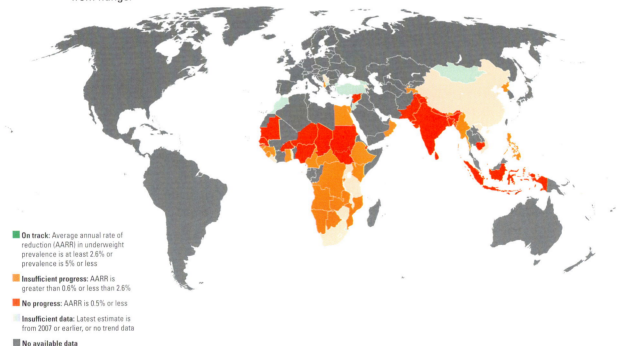

■ **On track:** Average annual rate of reduction (AARR) in underweight prevalence is at least 2.6% or prevalence is 5% or less

■ **Insufficient progress:** AARR is greater than 0.6% or less than 2.6%

■ **No progress:** AARR is 0.5% or less

■ **Insufficient data:** Latest estimate is from 2007 or earlier, or no trend data

■ **No available data**

Note: The classifications for Brazil and India differ from standard MDG1 progress classification.

This map is stylized and not to scale. It does not reflect a position by UNICEF on the legal status of any country or territory or the delimitation of any frontiers. The dotted line between Jammu and Kashmir represents approximately the Line of Control agreed upon by India and Pakistan. The final status of Jammu and Kashmir has not yet been agreed upon by the Parties. The final boundary between the Republic of the Sudan and the Republic of South Sudan has not yet been determined.

Source: UNICEF Global Nutrition Database, 2012, based on MICS, DHS and other national surveys.

Underweight

Globally in 2011, an estimated 101 million children under 5 years of age were underweight, or approximately 16 per cent of children under 5. Underweight prevalence is highest in South Asia, which has a rate of 33 per cent, followed by sub-Saharan Africa, at 21 per cent. South Asia has 59 million underweight children, while sub-Saharan Africa has 30 million.

The prevalence of underweight children under age 5 is an indicator to measure progress towards MDG 1, which aims to halve the proportion of people who suffer from hunger between 1990 and 2015. Globally, underweight prevalence has declined, from 25 per cent in 1990 to 16 per cent today – a 37 per cent reduction. The greatest reductions have been achieved in Central and Eastern Europe and the Commonwealth of Independent States, where prevalence has declined by 87 per cent, and in East Asia and the Pacific, where it fell 73 per cent (as with stunting, driven largely in the latter region by reductions made in China). In other regions, progress remained slow; in sub-Saharan Africa underweight prevalence dropped by 26 per cent.

As of 2011, 30 countries were on track to meet the MDG 1 target, 25 countries had made insufficient progress and 12 countries had made no progress *(Figure 11)*. Of the 24 countries profiled in this report, only 8 are on track to achieve the MDG 1 target. While countries make progress towards the target by decreasing underweight prevalence, these declines may represent an accompanying transition towards a higher prevalence of overweight with persistent levels of stunting.

FIGURE 11 | MDG 1 progress: 30 countries 'on track' as of 2011

Country progress towards MDG 1 target to halve, between 1990 and 2015, the proportion of people who suffer from hunger

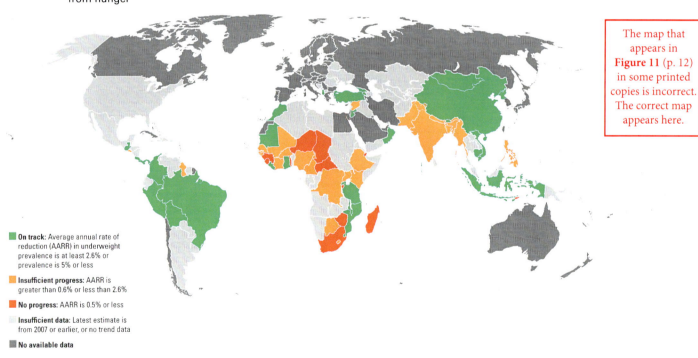

The map that appears in **Figure 11** (p. 12) in some printed copies is incorrect. The correct map appears here.

■ **On track:** Average annual rate of reduction (AARR) in underweight prevalence is at least 2.6% or prevalence is 5% or less

■ **Insufficient progress:** AARR is greater than 0.6% or less than 2.6%

■ **No progress:** AARR is 0.5% or less

□ **Insufficient data:** Latest estimate is from 2007 or earlier, or no trend data

■ **No available data**

Note: The classifications for Brazil and India differ from standard MDG1 progress classification.

This map is stylized and not to scale. It does not reflect a position by UNICEF on the legal status of any country or territory or the delimitation of any frontiers. The dotted line between Jammu and Kashmir represents approximately the Line of Control agreed upon by India and Pakistan. The final status of Jammu and Kashmir has not yet been agreed upon by the Parties. The final boundary between the Republic of the Sudan and the Republic of South Sudan has not yet been determined.

Source: UNICEF Global Nutrition Database, 2012, based on MICS, DHS and other national surveys.

Some countries have low underweight prevalence but unacceptably high stunting rates. For example, in Guatemala, Liberia, Malawi, Mozambique, Rwanda, the United Republic of Tanzania and Zambia, child underweight prevalence is lower than 20 per cent, while stunting prevalence remains above 40 per cent. Of the countries that are on track to achieve MDG 1, many still have high stunting rates. Cambodia, Guatemala, Liberia, Malawi, Mozambique, Rwanda and the United Republic of Tanzania have very high stunting prevalence (at least 40 per cent), while remaining on track to achieve MDG 1. Greater efforts should be made in these countries to prevent stunting, because the lower levels of underweight prevalence mask the continued existence of undernutrition during the crucial 1,000 days before the child's second birthday, including the mother's pregnancy.

Wasting

Moderate and severe wasting represents an acute form of undernutrition, and children who suffer from it face a markedly increased risk of death. Globally in 2011, 52 million children under 5 years of age were moderately or severely wasted, an 11 per cent decrease from the estimated figure of 58 million in 1990. More than 29 million children under 5, an estimated 5 per cent, suffered from severe wasting.[21]

The highest wasting prevalence is in South Asia, where approximately one in six children (16 per cent) is moderately or severely wasted. The burden of wasting is highest in India, which has more than 25 million wasted children. This exceeds the combined burden of the next nine high-burden countries (*Figure 12*).

In sub-Saharan Africa, nearly 1 in 10 children under the age of 5 (9 per cent) were wasted in 2011, a prevalence that has decreased about 10 per cent since 1990. Because of population growth, however, the region is now home to one third more wasted children than it was in 1990. The number of wasted children in sub-Saharan Africa as a proportion of the world's total has increased over the same period of time.

Countries like South Sudan, India, Timor-Leste, Sudan, Bangladesh and Chad have a very high prevalence of wasting – above 15 per cent. Of the 10 countries with the highest wasting prevalence, 7 also have rates for severe wasting above 5 per cent (*Figure 13*). Worldwide, of the 80 countries with available data, 23 have levels of wasting greater than 10 per cent (*Figure 14*).

While a significant number of the world's 52 million wasted children live in countries where cyclical food insecurity and protracted crises exacerbate their vulnerability, the majority reside in countries not affected by emergencies. In these countries factors such as frequent incidence of infectious diseases, inadequate caring capacity and social and cultural practices are the major factors that need to be addressed to reduce wasting.

FIGURE 12 **Wasting: Burden estimates in the 10 most affected countries**

Number of children under age 5 who are moderately or severely wasted

Ranked by burden (2011)	Country	Year	Wasting (%, moderate or severe)	Wasting (%, severe)	Number of wasted children, 2011 (moderate or severe, thousands)
1	India	2005–2006	20	6	25,461
2	Nigeria	2008	14	7	3,783
3	Pakistan	2011	15	6	3,339
4	Indonesia	2010	13	6	2,820
5	Bangladesh	2011	16	4	2,251
6	China	2010	3	–	1,891
7	Ethiopia	2011	10	3	1,156
8	Democratic Republic of the Congo	2010	9	3	1,024
9	Sudan	2010	16	5	817
10	Philippines	2008*	7	–	769

*Data differ from the standard definition or refer to only part of a country.

Source: UNICEF Global Nutrition Database, 2012, based on MICS, DHS and other national surveys, 2007–2011, except for India.

FIGURE 13 | Wasting: Prevalence estimates in the 10 most affected countries

Percentage of children under age 5 who are moderately or severely wasted

Ranked by prevalence (2007–2011)	Country	Year	Wasting prevalence (%, moderate or severe)	Wasting prevalence (%, severe)	Number of wasted children, 2011 (moderate and severe, thousands)
1	South Sudan	2010	23	10	338
2	India	2005–2006	20	6	25,461
3	Timor-Leste	2009–2010	19	7	38
4	Sudan	2010	16	5	817
5	Bangladesh	2011	16	4	2,251
6	Chad	2010	16	6	320
7	Pakistan	2011	15	6	3,339
8	Sri Lanka	2006–2007	15	3	277
9	Nigeria	2008	14	7	3,783
10	Indonesia	2010	13	6	2,820

Source: UNICEF Global Nutrition Database, 2012, based on MICS, DHS and other national surveys, 2007–2011, except for India.

FIGURE 14 | Prevalence of wasting is high in sub-Saharan Africa and South Asia

Percentage of children under age 5 who are moderately or severely wasted

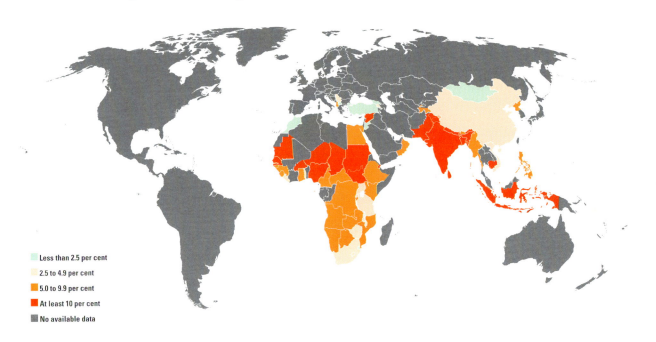

- Less than 2.5 per cent
- 2.5 to 4.9 per cent
- 5.0 to 9.9 per cent
- At least 10 per cent
- No available data

Note: Data are from 2007 to 2011, except for India.

This map is stylized and not to scale. It does not reflect a position by UNICEF on the legal status of any country or territory or the delimitation of any frontiers. The dotted line between Jammu and Kashmir represents approximately the Line of Control agreed upon by India and Pakistan. The final status of Jammu and Kashmir has not yet been agreed upon by the Parties. The final boundary between the Republic of the Sudan and the Republic of South Sudan has not yet been determined.

Source: UNICEF Global Nutrition Database, 2012, based on MICS, DHS and other national surveys, 2007–2011.

Overweight

Rates of overweight continue to rise across all regions. Overweight was once associated mainly with high-income countries, but in 2011, 69 per cent of the global burden of overweight children under 5 years old were in low- and middle-income countries. However, the prevalence of overweight remains higher in high-income countries (8 per cent) than in low-income countries (4 per cent).

Globally, an estimated 43 million children under 5 years of age are overweight, or 7 per cent of children under 5 years old. In 2011, approximately 10 million children in sub-Saharan Africa and 7 million in East Asia and the Pacific were overweight. There has been a substantial increase in the numbers of overweight children in these regions over the past two decades, contributing to an increase of around 50 per cent globally from 28 million children in 1990.

Prevalence estimates have more than doubled since 1990 in sub-Saharan Africa (from 3 per cent in 1990 to 7 per cent in 2011), meaning that more than three times as many children are affected today. A similar trend in estimates of child overweight has been observed in the Middle East and North Africa region.

FIGURE 15	Countries with overweight prevalence estimates of 10% or more

Percentage and number of children under age 5 who are overweight (including obese)

Ranked by prevalence (2007–2011)	Country	Year	Overweight* (%, including obese)	Number of overweight children, 2011 (including obese, thousands)
1	Albania	2008–2009	23	48
2	Libya	2007	22	160
3	Egypt	2008	21	1,864
4	Georgia	2009	20	51
5	Syrian Arab Republic	2009	18	438
6	Armenia	2010	17	38
7	Indonesia	2010	14	2,968
8	Sao Tome and Principe	2008–2009	12	3
9	Botswana	2007–2008	11	26
10	Swaziland	2010	11	17
11	Morocco	2010–2011	11	326
12	Nigeria	2008	11	2,858
13	Sierra Leone	2010	10	100

* By comparison, an estimated 12 per cent of children aged 2 to 5 years were overweight in the United States (NHANES 2009–2010).

Source: UNICEF Global Nutrition Database, 2012, based on MICS, DHS and other national surveys, 2007–2011.

Low birthweight

The World Health Assembly has set a new target to reduce low birthweight by 30 per cent between 2010 and 2025. In 2011, more than 20 million infants, an estimated 15 per cent globally, were born with low birthweight (*Figure 16*). India alone accounts for one third of the global burden. South Asia has by far the greatest regional incidence of low birthweight, with one in four newborns weighing less than 2,500 grams at birth (*Figure 17*).

The incidence of low birthweight exceeds 20 per cent in India, Mauritania, Nauru, Pakistan, and the Philippines, and in sub-Saharan Africa the incidence is greater than 10 per cent. More than 50 per cent of the global burden of low birthweight is attributed to 5 of the 24 countries profiled in this report.

One of the major challenges in measuring incidence of low birthweight is the fact that, as of 2011, more than half of the world's children had not been weighed at birth. This reflects a lack of appropriate newborn care and also presents a challenge to accurately estimating low birthweight incidence.

Methods have been developed to adjust for the problem of underreporting of birthweight, yet the rates are still likely to underestimate the true magnitude of the problem.

FIGURE 16 **Five countries account for more than half of the global low birthweight burden**

Number of infants weighing less than 2,500 grams at birth

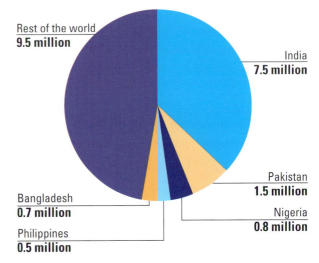

Rest of the world
9.5 million

India
7.5 million

Pakistan
1.5 million

Nigeria
0.8 million

Bangladesh
0.7 million

Philippines
0.5 million

Source: UNICEF Global Nutrition Database, 2012, based on MICS, DHS and other national surveys, 2007–2011, except for India.

FIGURE 17 **Low birthweight incidence is highest in South Asia**

Percentage of infants weighing less than 2,500 grams at birth

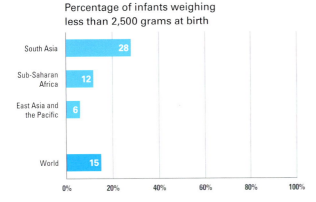

South Asia 28
Sub-Saharan Africa 12
East Asia and the Pacific 6
World 15

Percentage of infants not weighed at birth

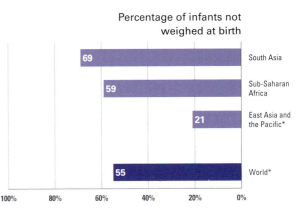

South Asia 69
Sub-Saharan Africa 59
East Asia and the Pacific* 21
World* 55

* Excludes China.

Source: UNICEF Global Nutrition Database, 2012, based on MICS, DHS and other national surveys, 2007–2011, except for India.

Chapter 4

INTERVENTIONS TO ADDRESS STUNTING AND OTHER FORMS OF UNDERNUTRITION

Nutrition-specific interventions are actions that have a direct impact on the prevention and treatment of undernutrition, in particular during the 1,000 days covering pregnancy and the child's first two years. These interventions should be complemented by broader, nutrition-sensitive approaches that have an indirect impact on nutrition status. Equity considerations in nutrition programming are particularly important, as stunting and other forms of undernutrition afflict the most vulnerable populations.

Nutrition-specific interventions

Promoting optimal nutrition practices, meeting micronutrient requirements and preventing and treating severe acute malnutrition are key goals for nutrition programming *(Figure 18)*. The 2009 *Tracking Progress on Child and Maternal Nutrition* report summarized the evidence base for nutrition-specific interventions. Taking a life-cycle approach, the activities fall broadly into the following categories:

- Maternal nutrition and prevention of low birthweight

- Infant and young child feeding (IYCF)
  - Breastfeeding, with early initiation (within one hour of birth) and continued exclusive breastfeeding for the first six months followed by continued breastfeeding up to 2 years

  - Safe, timely, adequate and appropriate complementary feeding from 6 months onwards

- Prevention and treatment of micronutrient deficiencies

- Prevention and treatment of severe acute malnutrition

- Promotion of good sanitation practices and access to clean drinking water

- Promotion of healthy practices and appropriate use of health services

Key proven practices, services and policy interventions for the prevention and treatment of stunting and other forms of undernutrition throughout the life cycle

ADOLESCENCE > PREGNANCY	BIRTH	0–5 MONTHS	6–23 MONTHS
• Improved use of locally available foods	• Early initiation of breastfeeding within one hour of delivery (including colostrum)	• Exclusive breastfeeding	• Timely introduction of adequate, safe and appropriate complementary feeding
• Food fortification, including salt iodization		• Appropriate infant feeding practices for HIV-exposed infants, and ARV	• Continued breastfeeding
• Micronutrient supplementation and deworming	• Appropriate infant feeding practices for HIV-exposed infants, and antivirals (ARV)	• Vitamin A supplementation in first eight weeks after delivery	• Appropriate infant feeding practices for HIV-exposed infants, and ARV
• Fortified food supplements for undernourished mothers		• Multi-micronutrient supplementation	• Micronutrient supplementation, including vitamin A, multi-micronutrients; zinc treatment for diarrhoea; deworming
• Antenatal care, including HIV testing		• Improved use of locally available foods, fortified foods, micronutrient supplementation/home fortification for undernourished women	• Community-based management of severe acute malnutrition; management of moderate acute malnutrition
			• Food fortification, including salt iodization
			• Prevention and treatment of infectious disease; hand washing with soap and improved water and sanitation practices
			• Improved use of locally available foods, fortified foods, micronutrient supplementation/home fortification for undernourished women, hand washing with soap

Note: Blue refers to interventions for women of reproductive age and mothers. Black refers to interventions for young children.

Source: Policy and guideline recommendations based on UNICEF, WHO and other United Nations agencies, Bhutta, Zulfiqar A., et al., 'Maternal and Child Undernutrition 3: What works? Interventions for maternal and child undernutrition and survival', *Lancet*, vol. 371, no. 9610, February 2008, pp. 417–440.

Maternal nutrition

Nutritional status before and during pregnancy influences maternal and child outcomes. Optimal child development requires adequate nutrient intake, provision of supplements as needed and prevention of disease. It also requires protection from stress factors such as cigarette smoke, narcotic substances, environmental pollutants and psychological stress.[22] Maternal malnutrition leads to poor foetal growth and low birthweight.

Interventions to improve maternal nutrient intake include supplementation with iron, folic acid or multiple micronutrients and provision of food and other supplements where necessary. Compared to iron-folic acid supplementation alone, supplementation with multiple micronutrients during pregnancy has been found to reduce low birthweight by about 10 per cent in low-income countries.[23] Adequate intake of folic acid and iodine around conception and of iron and iodine during pregnancy are important, especially for development of the infant's nervous system.

Among undernourished women, balanced protein-energy supplementation has been found effective in reducing the prevalence of low birthweight.[24] The use of lipid-based supplements for pregnant women in emergency settings is being studied as a way to improve child growth and development.[25]

Many interventions to promote maternal health and foetal growth are delivered by the health system and through community-based programmes. Antenatal care visits should be used to promote optimal nutrition and deliver specific interventions, such as malaria prophylaxis and treatment and deworming. Community-based education and communication programmes can encourage appropriate behaviours to improve nutrition. However, while 81 per cent of pregnant women benefit from at least one antenatal visit globally,[26] the coverage of specific interventions and the quality of antenatal care are variable.

Beyond such specific interventions, other relevant interventions include preventing pregnancy during adolescence, delaying age of marriage, preventing unwanted or unplanned pregnancy and overcoming sociocultural barriers to healthy practices and health-care seeking.

Infant and young child feeding

Optimal IYCF practices include initiating breastfeeding within one hour of birth, exclusive breastfeeding for the first six months of life and continued breast-feeding up to the age of 2 and beyond, together with safe, age-appropriate feeding of solid, semi-solid and soft food starting at 6 months of age.

Two practices together – ensuring optimal breastfeeding in the first year and complementary feeding practices – could prevent almost one fifth of deaths of children under 5 years of age.[27] Studies suggest that optimal breastfeeding improves brain development.[28] Breastfeeding may also protect against cardiovascular risk factors, although it is not yet clear whether this is the case in low- and middle-income settings.[29]

Nutrition programming in this area continues to receive insufficient attention, despite the well-established benefits of age-appropriate IYCF prac-tices. Valuable lessons from programming experiences have led to changes to IYCF strategies.[30] A compre-hensive, multi-pronged approach is needed, with both cross-cutting and targeted strategies at community, health system and national levels *(Figure 19)*.

Early initiation of breastfeeding
Several studies have demonstrated that early initiation of breastfeeding reduces the risk of neo-natal mortality.[31] Colostrum, the rich milk produced by the mother during the first few days after delivery, provides essential nutrients as well as antibodies to boost the baby's immune system, thus reducing the likelihood of death in the neonatal period. Beyond saving lives, early initiation of breastfeeding pro-motes stronger uterine contractions, reducing the likelihood of uterine bleeding. It also reduces the risk of hypothermia, improves bonding between mother and child and promotes early milk production.

Fewer than half of newborns globally are put to the breast within the first hour of birth *(Figure 20)*, though early initiation of breastfeeding is higher in least-developed countries (52 per cent in 2011). Breastfeeding is initiated within one hour of birth for fewer newborns in South Asia than in any other region (39 per cent in 2011). Sub-Saharan Africa leads coverage of early initiation of breastfeeding;

48 per cent of newborns are breastfed within one hour of birth. This is due to the high coverage in Eastern and Southern Africa of 56 per cent.[32]

FIGURE 19 | **Key components and interventions of an infant and young child feeding strategy**

Legislation
- Marketing of breastmilk substitutes
- Maternity protection

Skilled support by the health system
- Curriculum development for IYCF
- IYCF counselling and other support services
- Capacity development for health providers
- Institutionalization of the Baby-Friendly Hospital Initiative

Community-based counselling and support
- Established community-based integrated IYCF counselling services
- Mother support groups

Communication
- Communication for behaviour and social change

Additional complementary feeding options
- Improving the quality of complementary foods through locally available ingredients
- Increasing agricultural production
- Provision of nutrition supplements and foods
- Social protection schemes

IYCF in difficult circumstances
- HIV and infant feeding
- IYCF in emergencies

Source: Adapted from *Programming Guide: Infant and young child feeding*, UNICEF, 2011.

FIGURE 20 | **Globally, less than 40 per cent of infants are exclusively breastfed**

Percentage of children worldwide put to the breast within one hour of delivery; exclusively breastfed; both breastfed and receiving complementary foods; and continuing to breastfeed at specified ages

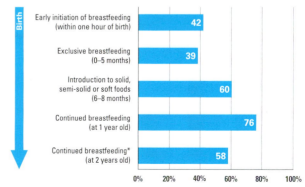

* Excludes China.

Source: UNICEF Global Nutrition Database, 2012, based on MICS, DHS and other national surveys, 2007–2011.

Exclusive breastfeeding

Exclusive breastfeeding in the first six months of life saves lives. During this period, an infant who is not breastfed is more than 14 times more likely to die from all causes than an exclusively breastfed infant.[33] Infants who are exclusively breastfed are less likely to die from diarrhoea and pneumonia, the two leading killers of children under 5.[34] Moreover, many other benefits are associated with exclusive breastfeeding for both mother and infant, including prevention of growth faltering.[35]

Globally 39 per cent of infants less than 6 months of age were exclusively breastfed in 2011 *(Figure 20)*. Some 76 per cent of infants continued to be breastfed at 1 year of age, while only 58 per cent continued through the recommended duration of up to two years. The regions with the highest exclusive breastfeeding rates of infants under 6 months old were Eastern and Southern Africa (52 per cent) and South Asia (47 per cent), with similar rates in least-developed countries as a whole. However, coverage is lowest in sub-Saharan Africa, with 37 per cent of infants less than 6 months of age exclusively breastfed in 2011. This is due largely to the low rate in West and Central Africa (25 per cent) compared to Eastern and Southern Africa (52 per cent).[36]

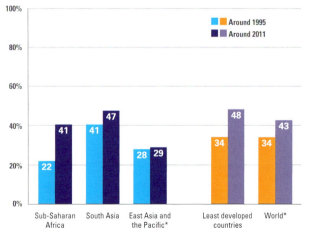
FIGURE 22 **Many countries have increased rates of exclusive breastfeeding**

Percentage of infants exclusively breastfed (0–5 months), by country, around 1995 and around 2011

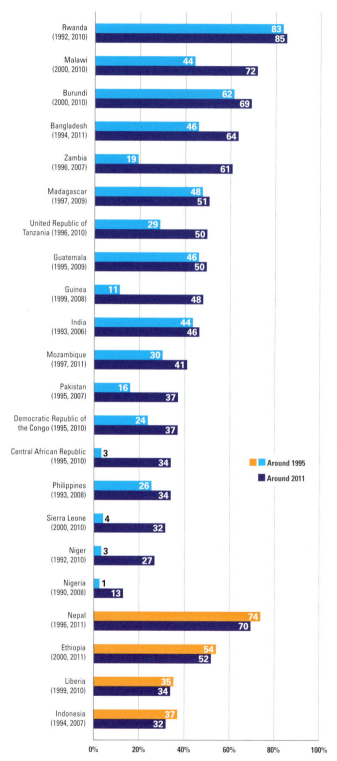

Note: The countries in this figure are profiled beginning on page 55 of this report.

Source: UNICEF Global Nutrition Database, 2012, based on MICS, DHS and other national surveys.

Rates of exclusive breastfeeding have increased by more than 20 per cent, from 34 per cent around 1995 to 43 per cent around 2011 *(Figure 21)*. It is particularly encouraging to note the nearly 50 per cent increase in exclusive breastfeeding rates in sub-Saharan Africa, from 22 per cent to 41 per cent during this period. Progress has also been made in least developed countries, where exclusive breastfeeding rates increased by nearly one third, from 34 per cent to 48 per cent.

Among 50 countries with available trend data, the majority (40 countries) have posted gains in exclusive breastfeeding rates since 1995.[37] Eighteen of these countries experienced increases of 20 per cent or more, illustrating that substantial improvement can be made and sustained through implementation of comprehensive, at-scale strategies. Most of the countries featured in this report have observed improvements in exclusive breastfeeding *(Figure 22)*. However, some countries (e.g., Chad, Cameroon and Nigeria) still experience low rates of exclusive breastfeeding in parallel with high rates of stunting.

Complementary feeding

Studies have shown that feeding with appropriate, adequate and safe complementary foods from the age of 6 months onwards leads to better health and growth outcomes.[38] Breastmilk remains an important source of nutrients, and it is recommended that breastfeeding continue until children reach 2 years of age. In vulnerable populations especially, good complementary feeding practices have been shown to reduce stunting markedly and rapidly.[39] However, children may not receive safe and appropriate complementary foods at the right age, may not be fed at the right frequency or may receive food of inadequate quality.[40] The problem of poor quality of complementary food has been underemphasized in nutrition programming for quite some time.[41]

BOX 4

Seizing opportunities to improve breastfeeding through existing health service delivery

Across the continuum of care, several opportunities exist to synergize interventions and reinforce messaging to improve health and nutrition. For example, during antenatal care and at the time of delivery, women can be counselled about the benefits of early initiation of exclusive breastfeeding.

While almost two thirds of births globally were attended by a skilled professional in 2011, less than one half of infants were put to the breast within an hour of birth. This disjuncture reveals a missed opportunity to assist women with breastfeeding at a time when they are already in contact with the health system.

Within sub-Saharan Africa, the proportion of infants delivered by a skilled health professional and put to the breast within one hour of birth varies by region. In West and Central Africa, while the proportion of births attended by a skilled professional is greater than in Eastern and Southern Africa, the rate of early initiation of breastfeeding is lower *(Figure 23)*. More efforts are needed to improve the content and quality of maternal care by training health-care providers and strengthening systems to effectively support optimal breastfeeding practices. This, together with improving access to health care, can help integrate nutrition into existing health delivery platforms and maximize the benefits of synergy.

FIGURE 23 | **Contact with the health system is not resulting in early initiation of breastfeeding**

Percentage of pregnant mothers with at least one antenatal care visit with a skilled health professional; percentage of births attended by a skilled health professional; and percentage of infants who were put to the breast within one hour of birth

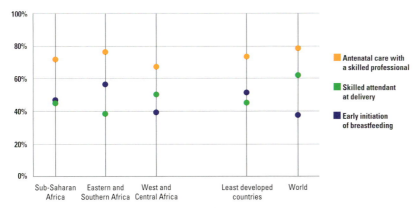

- ■ Antenatal care with a skilled professional
- ■ Skilled attendant at delivery
- ■ Early initiation of breastfeeding

Note: Regional analysis based on a subset of 54 countries with available data for each indicator. Regional estimates are presented only where adequate population coverage is met.

Source: UNICEF Global Nutrition Database, 2012, based on MICS, DHS and other national surveys, 2007–2011, except for India.

Key principles guide programming for complementary feeding.[42] They include education to improve caregiver practices; increasing energy density and/or nutrient bioavailability of complementary foods; providing complementary foods, with or without added micronutrients; and fortifying complementary foods, either centrally or through home fortification including use of multiple micronutrient powder (MNP), in each case paying greater attention to food-insecure populations.

Globally, only 60 per cent of children aged 6 to 8 months receive solid, semi-solid or soft foods, highlighting deficiencies in the timely introduction of complementary foods. Of the 24 countries profiled in this report, only 8 had recent data reflecting both the frequency and quality of complementary feeding for children aged 6 to 23 months (Figure 24).

'Minimum acceptable diet' is a composite indicator that incorporates both meal frequency and dietary diversity. Among the profiled countries, the percentage of children receiving a minimum acceptable diet ranged from 24 per cent in Nepal to just 4 per cent in Ethiopia. Urgent attention is needed to monitor and improve the quantity and quality of complementary feeding.

FIGURE 24 | **Complementary feeding in eight countries**

Percentage of breastfed and non-breastfed children aged 6–23 months receiving minimum acceptable diet, minimum dietary diversity, and minimum meal frequency

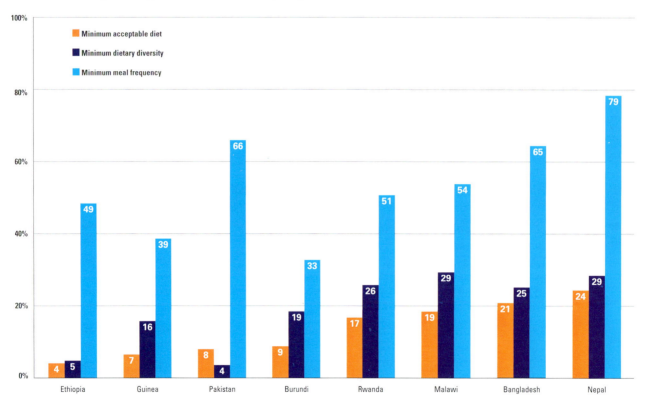

Note: The eight countries selected were those profiled in this report with available data on complementary feeding indicators.

Minimum meal frequency refers to the percentage of children aged 6–23 months who received solid, semi-solid or soft foods the minimum number of times or more (for breastfed children, minimum is defined as two times for infants 6–8 months and three times for children 9–23 months; for non-breastfed children, minimum is defined as four times for children 6–23 months); minimum dietary diversity refers to the percentage of children aged 6–23 months who received foods from four or more food groups; and minimum acceptable diet refers to the percentage of children aged 6–23 months who received a minimum acceptable diet both in terms of frequency and quality, apart from breastmilk.

Source: UNICEF Global Nutrition Database, 2012, based on MICS, DHS and other national surveys, 2010–2012.

Prevention and treatment of micronutrient deficiencies

Micronutrient deficiencies, including deficiencies of vitamin A, iron, iodine, zinc and folic acid, are common among women and children in low- and middle-income countries. Ensuring adequate micronutrient status in women of reproductive age, pregnant women and children improves the health of expectant mothers, the growth and development of unborn children, and the survival and physical and mental development of children up to 5 years old.

Programmes to address micronutrient deficiencies include delivery of supplements to specific vulnerable groups, home fortification of complementary food for children aged 6 to 23 months and fortification of staple foods and condiments.

Vitamin A supplementation

Globally, one in three preschool-aged children and one in six pregnant women are deficient in vitamin A due to inadequate dietary intake (1995–2005 data).[43] The highest prevalence remains in Africa and South-East Asia. Vitamin A is necessary to support immune system response, and children who are deficient face a higher risk of dying from infectious diseases such as measles and diarrhoea. Vitamin A supplementation delivered periodically to children aged 6 to 59 months has been shown to be highly effective in reducing mortality from all causes in countries where vitamin A deficiency is a public health problem.

In many developing countries, especially where coverage by the routine health system is weak, vitamin A supplements are delivered to children during integrated health events, such as child health days. These events allow for the periodic delivery of key child survival interventions including immunization, deworming and mosquito net provision. Particularly in sub-Saharan Africa, countries that have adopted this approach have managed to sustain high coverage of vitamin A supplementation even in hard to reach areas.

Globally, three in four children (75 per cent) aged 6 to 59 months received two doses of vitamin A in 2011, fully protecting them against vitamin A deficiency (Figure 25). Coverage of vitamin A supplementation was highest in East Asia and the Pacific

(85 per cent; excluding China for lack of data) and West and Central Africa (83 per cent). Nearly half of countries reporting these data in 2011 did not reach the 80 per cent coverage target.

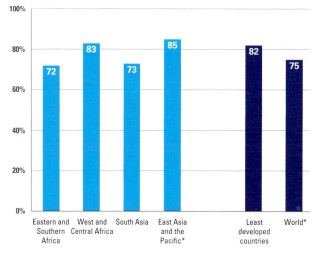

FIGURE 25 **Vitamin A supplementation reaches more than 80 per cent of young children in least developed countries**

Percentage of children aged 6–59 months who received two doses of vitamin A in 2011

* Excludes China.

Source: UNICEF Global Nutrition Databases, 2012. Regional estimates are presented only where adequate population coverage is met.

Iron supplementation

Iron deficiency predominantly affects children, adolescents and menstruating and pregnant women. Globally, the most significant contributor to the onset of anaemia is iron deficiency. Consequences of iron deficiency include reduced school performance in children and decreased work productivity in adults. Anaemia is most prevalent in Africa and Asia, especially among poor populations. Global estimates from the WHO database suggest that about 42 per cent of pregnant women and 47 per cent of preschool-aged children suffer from anaemia.[44]

In most countries profiled in this report, less than one third of women received adequate iron-folic acid supplementation for more than 90 days during their last pregnancy.[45] Anaemia prevalence among preschool-aged children exceeds 40 per cent in almost all countries profiled in this report that have available data.

Universal salt iodization

Iodine deficiency is the most common cause of preventable mental impairment. Fortification of salt is widely used to avert consequences associated with this deficiency. Significant progress has been made in reducing the number of countries whose populations suffer mild to severe iodine deficiency, from 54 countries in 2003 to 32 in 2011. During this period the number of countries reaching adequate iodine intake increased by more than one third, from 43 to 69.

Globally, 75 per cent of households have adequately iodized salt (15 parts per million or more), but coverage varies considerably by region *(Figure 26)*. East Asia and the Pacific had the highest coverage, 87 per cent in 2011, and as a region had nearly reached the universal salt iodization target of 90 per cent. Coverage was lowest in sub-Saharan Africa, where less than half of households have adequately iodized salt. Coverage is generally higher among richer households than poorer households *(Figure 27)*.

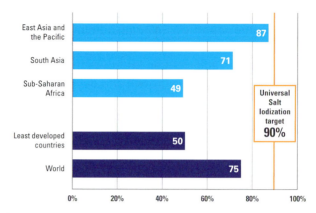

FIGURE 26 | **Globally, three out of four households consume adequately iodized salt**

Percentage of households with adequately iodized salt (15 ppm or more), 2007–2011

East Asia and the Pacific: 87
South Asia: 71
Sub-Saharan Africa: 49
Least developed countries: 50
World: 75

Universal Salt Iodization target **90%**

Source: UNICEF Global Nutrition Database, 2012, based on MICS, DHS and other national surveys, 2007–2011. Regional estimates are presented only where adequate population coverage is met.

FIGURE 27 | **Iodized salt consumption is more likely among the richest households than the poorest households**

Consumption of adequately iodized salt among the richest households compared to the poorest, in countries with available data

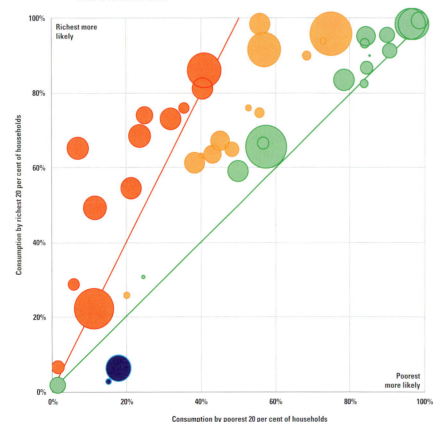

- ● Richest 20% more than twice as likely as poorest 20% (12 countries)
- ● Richest 20% more likely than poorest 20% (13 countries)
- ● Richest 20% equally as likely as poorest 20% (16 countries)
- ● Richest 20% less likely than poorest 20% (2 countries)

How to read this graph:
Each circle represents data from one country. The size of a circle is proportional to the size of the country's population. The horizontal axis represents the percentage of the poorest 20 per cent of households consuming adequately iodized salt, while the vertical axis represents the percentage of the richest 20 per cent of households. Circles along the green line represent countries in which the likelihood of consuming adequately iodized salt is similar among the richest and the poorest households. Circles above or below the green line suggest disparity. The closeness of circles to the upper-left corner indicates greater advantage for the richest households in that country (greater disadvantage for the poorest households).

Note: Based on 43 countries with available disparity data.

Source: UNICEF Global Nutrition Database, 2012, MICS, DHS and other national surveys, with additional analysis by UNICEF, 2006–2011.

One fifth of countries reporting in 2011 had reached the 90 per cent target of universal salt iodization.[46] Most had reached only 50 to 70 per cent coverage. Support of national salt iodization programmes is needed, along with advocacy to increase awareness among country policymakers about the need to eliminate iodine deficiency, private-public partnerships to assist salt producers with sustained iodization, and education of civil society to build demand for iodized salt.

Fortification of complementary foods, staple foods and condiments

Home fortification

Multiple micronutrient powders (MNPs) offer a low-cost, highly acceptable way to improve the quality of complementary foods. MNPs have been found highly effective in preventing iron deficiency and iron-deficiency anaemia. Combined with additional supplementary energy, protein and fats, MNPs have also been shown to improve child growth and development.[47]

Based on a global assessment carried out in 2011, some 22 countries, mostly in Asia and Latin America and the Caribbean, were implementing MNP interventions to improve the quality of complementary food. They reached over 12 million children in 2010, mainly by distributing MNPs through the public health system. Four countries are implementing national-scale programmes and 17 countries are working to scale up to a national level. Further expansion is taking place, mainly in Africa and South-East Asia.[48]

Large-scale fortification

Adding micronutrients to staple foods, complementary foods and condiments in factories and other production sites is a cost-effective way to improve the micronutrient status of populations. For example, flour is commonly fortified with iron, zinc, folic acid and other B vitamins such as thiamine, riboflavin, niacin and vitamin B12. As of December 2012, wheat flour fortification is mandated by law in 75 countries compared with only 33 countries in 2004. The amount of flour currently fortified represents about 30 per cent of the global production of wheat flour from industrial mills.[49]

Prevention and treatment of severe acute malnutrition

Children with severe acute malnutrition (SAM) are nine times more likely to die than children who are well-nourished.[50] Children who are wasted, have highly variable weight for height or experience negative changes in weight for height, are at a higher risk for linear growth retardation and stunting.[51]

While prevention is the first step towards management of SAM, once it occurs, urgent action is needed to minimize complications and avoid the risk of death. It is increasingly recognized that SAM is a problem not only in emergency contexts but also in non-emergency settings.

Community-based management has proven to be successful in treating acute malnutrition[52] and was officially endorsed by the United Nations in 2007. It decentralizes the management of SAM, making it easier to reach and treat children in their communities. It involves early detection of children with SAM with treatment in the community, timely referral to inpatient care for those who need it and subsequent follow-up in the community. Multiple partners have supported this approach in both emergency and non-emergency settings by guiding policy change, providing technical support and making commitments to provide therapeutic supplies. Using this approach, more than 75 per cent of treated children are expected to recover. In addition, more children have access to treatment because hospitalization is not required for the majority of cases.[53]

Globally in 2011, an estimated 2 million children under 5 were admitted for treatment of SAM – compared with just over 1 million reported during 2009.[54] This increase in reported admissions is not only indicative of improved access to SAM management, but also reflects improved national reporting. More than 80 per cent of the 2 million children treated were in sub-Saharan Africa. Five countries (Ethiopia, Niger, Somalia, Pakistan and the Democratic Republic of the Congo) accounted for a little more than 1 million admissions – roughly 56 per cent of all admissions globally (Figure 28).

Key strategies to expand access to quality treatment of SAM include creating national policies to help governments accelerate and sustain scale-up, building national capacities and strengthening systems to support SAM scale-up, and integrating SAM into other health and nutrition activities.

FIGURE 28	Five countries account for more than half of admissions for treatment of severe acute malnutrition

Number of reported cases admitted for treatment of SAM in 2011

Country	Cases admitted for treatment of SAM
Ethiopia	302,000
Niger	299,000
Somalia	167,000
Pakistan	157,000
Democratic Republic of the Congo	157,000
Total	**1,082,000**

Note: Figures are presented to the nearest 1,000. There is no standardized system of national reporting, therefore the mode of each country's data collection differs (whether based on health facilities with functional services for SAM or numbers of implementing partners submitting reports). Also note that while Niger, Somalia and Pakistan received 100 per cent of expected reports for 2011, Ethiopia and the Democratic Republic of the Congo indicated receiving 80 per cent of expected reports.

Source: UNICEF Global Nutrition Database, based on Global SAM Update, 2012.

Water, sanitation and hygiene and access to health services

Repeated episodes of diarrhoea, intestinal infestation with nematode worms and possibly tropical or environmental enteropathy (in which faecal contamination causes changes to the intestines affecting permeability and absorption) can impede nutrient absorption and diminish appetite, resulting in stunting and other forms of undernutrition.[55]

Improving water, sanitation and hygiene as well as housing and access to and use of health services can promote healthy environments and reduce the prevalence of infectious diseases,[56] and key interventions implemented at scale can reduce undernutrition. These include immunization, improving sanitation by creating environments free of open defecation, hand washing with soap, access to clean drinking water, use of oral rehydration salts and therapeutic zinc to treat diarrhoea, prevention (with insecticide-treated mosquito nets) and treatment of malaria, and treatment of pneumonia with antibiotics. Ongoing research is needed to help quantify the effect and the effectiveness of interventions in different settings.

Community-based approaches

Scale-up of integrated, community-based nutrition programmes linked with health, water and sanitation, and other relevant interventions is a priority strategy that can bring measurable improvements in children's nutritional status, survival and development. Community support can include providing services such as counselling, support and communication on IYCF; screening for acute malnutrition and follow-up of malnourished children; deworming; and delivering vitamin A and micronutrient supplements. Synergizing nutrition-specific interventions with other early child development interventions at the community level is also important for holistically promoting early child development and reducing inequalities.

Communication for behaviour and social change

Based on formative research on the barriers to and the facilitators of good nutrition, communication for behaviour and social change can promote behaviour change in communities, raise awareness about nutrition services and stimulate shifts in social norms in order to improve the enabling environment for good nutrition in communities.

Nutrition-sensitive approaches

Nutrition-sensitive approaches involve other sectors in indirectly addressing the underlying causes of undernutrition. There is less evidence for the impact of nutrition-sensitive approaches than for direct nutrition-specific interventions, in part because they are hard to measure. However, policies and programming in agriculture, education, social protection and poverty reduction are important for realizing nutrition goals. Achieving nutrition-sensitive development requires multi-sectoral coordination and cooperation with many stakeholders, which has historically been challenging in nutrition. Agriculture and social protection programmes are discussed in more detail below.

Agriculture

Recently, attention has increasingly been paid to improving synergies and linkages between agriculture and nutrition and health, in both the programmatic and the research communities.[57]

The global agricultural system is currently producing enough food to feed the world, but access to adequate, affordable, nutritious food is more challenging. Improving dietary diversity by increasing production of nutritious foods is achievable, particularly in rural populations. It is done by producing nutrient-dense foods, such as fruits and vegetables, fish, livestock, milk and eggs; increasing the nutritional content of foods through crop biofortification and post-harvest fortification; improving storage and preservation of foods to cover 'lean' seasons; and educating people about nutrition and diet. In several settings these types of interventions have been shown to improve dietary patterns and intake of specific micronutrients, either directly or by increasing household income. However, the impact on stunting, wasting and micronutrient deficiencies is less clear.[58]

More effort is needed to align the pursuit of food security with nutrition security and improved nutritional outcomes.

Social protection

Social protection involves policies and programmes that protect people against vulnerability, mitigate the impacts of shocks, improve resilience and support people whose livelihoods are at risk. Safety nets are a type of social protection that provides or substitutes for income: Targeted cash transfers and food access-based approaches are the two main categories of safety nets intended to avert starvation and reduce undernutrition among the most vulnerable populations. Food-based safety nets are designed to ensure livelihoods (such as public works employment paid in food), increase purchasing power (through food stamps, coupons or vouchers) and relieve deprivation (by providing food directly to households or individuals).

While social safety net programmes operate in at least a dozen countries, evidence indicating that these programmes have improved child nutritional status

is still limited.[59] A review of evaluations of conditional cash transfer programmes showed an impact on stunting in two of five studies, the Familias en Acción programme in Colombia and the Oportunidades programme in Mexico. Of the three unconditional cash transfer programmes, two (South African Child Support Grants and Ecuador's Bono Solidario) reduced stunting.[60] More research and evidence is needed on the long-term outcomes of these programmes and how they can be better targeted, how long they are needed and with what interventions. But social safety net programmes may be one way to ensure more equitable nutrition-sensitive development if they are aligned with local and national needs and an understanding of capacity, resources and timeliness aspects in scaling up.

Maintaining the focus on equity

As emphasized throughout this report, maintaining a focus on equity is particularly important, because stunting and other forms of undernutrition are concentrated among the most disadvantaged in society.

Undernutrition is inextricably linked with poverty. Equity-focused nutrition programming and other development strategies can effectively address the inequalities caused by poverty and the forms of exclusion that exist among groups and individuals.

For biological reasons, women and children are more vulnerable to nutritional deficiencies; special efforts are therefore needed to address the biological and social inequities that affect them. Women's low education levels, unequal social status and limited decision-making power can negatively influence the nutrition status of their children, as well as their own. Improving access to education and creating opportunities for both girls and boys, and their families, will confer many benefits in terms of nutritional status and child development.

Creating an enabling environment that targets the needs of vulnerable people is crucial. Since inequalities in nutritional status have a long-lasting, intergenerational impact on a country's physical, social and economic well-being, the response by communities and governments has implications for the nation's pursuit of equitable development.

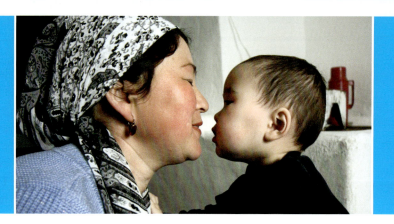

Chapter **5**

IT CAN BE DONE: SUCCESS STORIES IN SCALING UP NUTRITION

Nutrition programming in diverse countries has shed light on the factors that lead to sustainable advances in a country's nutrition status. These elements of success include political commitment and strong government leadership; evidence-based nutrition policy; coordinated and collaborative partnerships across sectors; good technical capacity and programme design; sufficient resources to strengthen implementation; and mechanisms to increase stakeholder demand for nutrition programming. Also required is a robust monitoring and evaluation system that can be used to improve real-time programme implementation and demonstrate impact. As some of the following case studies illustrate, programmes that are targeted to specific populations and are able to maintain a strong equity focus help reduce inequalities in child nutritional status.

The successes presented here represent a broad range of contexts, reflecting the diversity and complexity of nutrition programming. The first six case studies focus on reducing stunting; the remaining five case studies cover specific programming aspects related to the management of severe acute malnutrition, infant and young child feeding, micronutrients and nutrition policy reform. Despite the challenges of nutrition programming, the countries featured here have achieved remarkable improvements in policies and programmes as well as in behaviour change and nutritional status – and, importantly, they have achieved them at scale.[61]

Ethiopia: Reducing undernutrition with national planning

Much of Ethiopia depends on rain-fed agriculture, making the population vulnerable to drought and food insecurity. Yet the country has managed to reduce under-five mortality and stunting over the past decade. Between 2000 and 2011, under-five mortality fell from an estimated 139 deaths per 1,000 live births to 77 per 1,000,[62] close to the MDG 4 target of 66 per 1,000. Rates of stunting among children under 5 also decreased during this period, from an estimated 57 per cent to 44 per cent.[63]

However, more than 5 million children remained stunted in 2011,[64] even though per capita gross national income in Ethiopia grew from US$130 in 2000 to US$400 in 2011.[65] Stunting existed across households both poor and rich, indicating that economic growth and food security alone were not sufficient to reduce child stunting.[66]

Key strategy: A strong safety net and a comprehensive plan

In 2008, the Government of Ethiopia launched a National Nutrition Programme (NNP), combining nutrition services into one comprehensive strategy. The NNP shifted the previous focus on food aid and humanitarian assistance and increased attention on comprehensive direct nutrition interventions addressing the immediate and underlying causes of malnutrition, especially at community level. This programme is enhanced by Ethiopia's robust social protection strategies, including:

- A safety net programme covering more than 7 million people in the poorest areas of the country.

- An emergency response system and several programmes reaching populations in areas not covered by the safety net.

- Scaling up of community nutrition programmes, contributing to improved infant feeding practices.

- Micronutrient supplementation and treatment of SAM.

- A package of free health services, providing insecticide-treated mosquito nets, pneumonia treatment, family planning and support for treatment of acute diarrhoea.

This comprehensive NNP strategy is well aligned with the government's Food Security Strategy. One element of this is the Productive Safety Net Programme, introduced in 2005, which hires people for public works or provides food or cash transfers to families. The programme has had a positive impact on addressing food insecurity, one of the underlying causes of stunting: Between 2006 and 2010, the number of months of food security increased significantly in covered areas, as did the number of meals children consumed during lean seasons.[67]

An important NNP component is the Community-Based Nutrition Programme, which concentrates on improving the nutritional status of children under age 2. The programme strengthens communities' capacity to assess undernutrition, understand the causes and actions needed, and improve use of family, community and external resources. Community health services deliver nutrition interventions through trained health extension workers. Since the programme began in 2008, coverage increased from 39 districts to 228 districts in 2012, with plans to expand further in 2013.

Ethiopia is also addressing SAM by strengthening community management, providing micronutrient supplementation through community health days, and promoting optimal infant and young child feeding.

Community-based nutrition interventions are integrated into health services through the Health Extension Programme. In existence at the launch of the NNP, it expanded to cover all rural communities in 2008, increasing primary-health-care coverage (including nutrition interventions) from 77 per cent of communities in 2004 to 92 per cent in 2010.[68] Evidence from evaluations suggests that services have improved and people have changed their behaviour.[69] In 2011, 71 per cent of children 6–59 months were fully protected against vitamin A deficiency with supplementation. Furthermore, 52 per cent of children 0–5 months were exclusively breastfed.

Looking forward

A revised NNP is expected to be released in late 2013, increasing the emphasis on multi-sectoral nutrition interventions. It will align with the Health Sector Development Plan, which provides an opportunity to further expand coverage of key nutrition and health services. The Community-Based Nutrition Programme is a strong vehicle for targeting interventions at community level. It can help to address inequalities in child nutritional status, but it needs to be scaled up nationally, with support from key partners. This will require more financing to support investment in health system capacity. The Government of Ethiopia has joined the SUN movement and is committed to increasing resources for the NNP and putting into place measures to align and accelerate actions to improve food security and nutrition. ■

Haiti: Expanding nutrition services in an emergency

The earthquake that struck Haiti in January 2010 affected around 3 million people, causing widespread devastation and exacerbating already challenging conditions. Assessments conducted immediately after the earthquake showed that about half of the households in the affected area – around 1.3 million people – were food insecure.[70] A survey conducted several months later found that at least 41 per cent of children aged 6–59 months were reported to have suffered an episode of illness, mainly diarrhoea, acute respiratory infections and fever – among the principal causes of death in children.[71] This situation raised the risk of death and malnutrition for infants, young children and pregnant and lactating women.

Despite this humanitarian crisis, the Government of Haiti and the international community together were able to provide a package of services to address the high burden of stunting among children less than 5 years old. Preliminary survey results indicate that prevalence fell from an estimated 29 per cent to 22 per cent between 2006 and 2012 (Figure 29).

FIGURE 29 | Stunting, underweight and wasting trends in Haiti, 2000–2012

Percentage of children under age 5 who are moderately or severely stunted, underweight or wasted

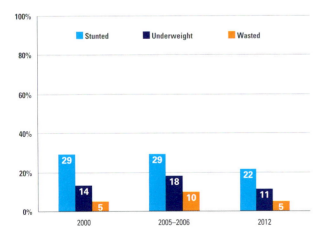

Source: Haiti Demographic and Health Surveys, 2000 and 2005–2006; Preliminary Demographic and Health Survey (pDHS), 2012.

Key strategy: Rapid expansion of basic health and nutrition services

A few months after the earthquake, the government developed the National Action Plan for Recovery and Redevelopment. Its rapid implementation shows that basic nutrition and health services can be expanded in the aftermath of an emergency and can dramatically improve the nutritional status of children. This progress in the face of extreme challenges resulted from a number of strategies, including:

- Food distribution and cash-for-work or cash transfers to buy food for the most affected and vulnerable households.

- Nutrition counselling in communities to increase exclusive breastfeeding and improve feeding practices.

- Micronutrient supplementation and growth monitoring and promotion.

- Integrated management of acute malnutrition.

- Community outreach to improve contacts with households and expand coverage of nutrition services.

In the year following the disaster, nutritious food, including ready-to-use therapeutic food, was distributed to about 4 million Haitians, and 900,000 received help through cash-for-work or cash transfers to ensure sufficient food consumption.[72] This led to a dramatic drop in the percentage of food-insecure households in earthquake-affected and other vulnerable areas, from 52 per cent in early 2010 to 39 per cent just four months later.[73]

Nutrition Counselling Points for Babies (PCNBs; Points de conseils de nutrition pour les bébés) set up in earthquake-affected areas empowered communities to combat malnutrition and improve IYCF practices. PCNBs, which came to be known as 'baby tents', also promoted early detection of malnutrition and access to treatment. During 2010 and 2011, more than 230,000 children and pregnant and breastfeeding mothers received services, including counselling on infant and young child feeding, micro-nutrient supplementation and growth monitoring and promotion, at about 200 PCNBs.[74]

This community outreach strategy contributed significantly to expanded coverage of nutrition interventions. Early initiation of breastfeeding increased from 44 per cent in 2006[75] to 64 per cent in 2012 as reported by the government;[76] in PCNB areas, 70 per cent of children younger than 6 months were exclusively breastfed in 2012, according to UNICEF estimates.[77] In 2010, more than 500,000 pregnant women received iron-folic acid and iodine supplements and more than 1 million children aged 6–59 months benefited from interventions to address micronutrient deficiencies. More than 15,000 children aged 6 to 59 months were admitted for treatment of SAM.[78] In addition, 31,050 long-lasting insecticide-treated mosquito nets were distributed in four of the most malaria-endemic areas and more than 11,300 latrines were provided.[79]

Looking forward

Haiti still faces many challenges, including the fact that around one in five children under 5 are stunted. The international community, which rallied around Haiti in the crisis, is phasing out its emergency support. This leaves Haiti with the critical task of providing basic health and nutrition services with insufficient qualified personnel and an infrastructure that is still recovering.

The government and its partners have begun working to build up the long-term capacity of the health system and communities. Haiti has joined the SUN movement, signalling its commitment to prioritize food and nutrition security and invest in direct nutrition interventions. A new national nutrition policy has recently been put in place to guide this process. ■

India: Improving nutrition governance to reduce child stunting in Maharashtra

More than 60 million children under 5 are stunted in India, comprising almost half the children in this age group. They represent an estimated one third of stunted children worldwide.[80] Even in Maharashtra, the wealthiest state in India, 39 per cent of children under age 2 were stunted in 2005–2006. But by 2012, according to a statewide nutrition survey, the prevalence of stunting had dropped to 23 per cent.[81] The state's determined actions and focus on service delivery contributed to this dramatic decline.

Key strategy: Building staff capacity to improve delivery of services

In 2005, in response to reports of child deaths from undernutrition in a number of districts, the state launched the Rajmata Jijau Mother-Child Health & Nutrition Mission. It was initially focused on five primarily tribal districts with the highest incidence of child undernutrition (Amravati, Gadchiroli, Nandurbar, Nasik and Thane). But after the National Family Health Survey of 2005–2006, the Mission's mandate was expanded to coordinate efforts to reduce child undernutrition throughout the state, an initiative of enormous significance given that Maharashtra is the second most populous state in India. The Mission was extended to 10 additional districts with a substantial concentration of tribal populations in 2006–2007 and finally to the remaining districts in 2008–2009.

The State Nutrition Mission began by working to improve the effectiveness of service delivery through the Integrated Child Development Services and the National Rural Health Mission, the national flagship programmes for child nutrition, health and development. Their focus was on filling vacancies in key personnel, particularly front-line workers and supervisors, and on improving their motivation and skills to deliver timely, high-quality services in communities. In the second five-year phase, beginning in 2011, more emphasis was placed on improving the nutrition of children under 2 and their mothers. This shift was made in response to global evidence about the critical 1,000-day window to prevent undernutrition in children.

In 2012, the Government of Maharashtra commissioned the first-ever statewide nutrition survey to assess progress and identify areas for future action. Results of this Comprehensive Nutrition Survey in Maharashtra indicated that prevalence of stunting in children under 2 was 23 per cent in 2012 – a decrease of 16 percentage points over a seven-year period.[82] Progress was associated with improvements in how children were fed, the care they and their mothers received, and the environments in which they lived. From 2005–2006 to 2012, the percentage of children 6 to 23 months old who were fed a required minimum number of times per day increased from 34 to 77 and the proportion of mothers who benefited from at least three antenatal visits during pregnancy increased from 75 to 90 per cent.[83]

The Maharashtra Nutrition Mission is tackling stunting among children under age 2 statewide by promoting more effective delivery of interventions through flagship programmes for child survival, growth and development. Four factors are seen as key to the state's success:

- Remaining focused: Efforts are concentrated on delivering evidence-based interventions for infants, young children and their mothers to prevent stunting while simultaneously addressing adolescent girls' nutrition, education and empowerment to improve the start in life for the next generation.

- Delivering at scale with equity: Efforts are made to combine services in facilities with outreach and community-based interventions to bring them closer to children under 2, adolescent girls and mothers. To ensure equity and impact, the focus is on the most vulnerable children, households, districts and divisions.

- Improving children's birthweight: The approach calls for monitoring pregnancy weight gain at every antenatal care visit and counselling and supporting mothers to gain adequate weight during pregnancy. In addition, all children are weighed at birth, and children born weighing below 2,500 grams are monitored to ensure they catch up.

- Coordinating and measuring for nutrition results across sectors: Planning and management are focused on nutrition results, and indicators of child nutrition are integrated across programmes and sectors. Another emphasis is on building strong monitoring and evaluation frameworks to measure programme performance.

Looking forward

The provisional results of the Maharashtra survey showed that in spite of more frequent meals, only 7 per cent of children 6–23 months old received a minimal acceptable diet in 2012. Too few children are being fed an adequately diverse diet rich in essential nutrients with the appropriate frequency to ensure their optimal physical growth and cognitive development. A statewide strategy to improve the quality of complementary foods and feeding and hygiene practices is essential to further reduce stunting levels and bring about far-reaching benefits. ∎

Nepal: Making steady progress for women and children

About one quarter of Nepal's people live below the national poverty line, and the country has emerged from a decade-long internal conflict that ended with a peace accord in 2006. Despite these challenges, Nepal has made impressive progress for human development over the past decade.

The proportion of people living on less than US$1.25 per day has fallen by half in seven years, from 53 per cent in 2003 to 25 per cent in 2010.[84] Under-five mortality has also decreased substantially since 2000, from 83 deaths per 1,000 live births to 48 per 1,000 in 2011.[85] Stunting prevalence among children under age 5 dropped from 57 per cent in 2001 to 41 per cent in 2011,[86] showing that even in difficult conditions, impressive gains can be made.

Key strategy: Community-based interventions to reduce child stunting

The success in reducing child stunting took place against a backdrop of economic growth and poverty reduction, but it was also driven by combining important health and nutrition strategies:

- Delivery of interventions through community-based programming facilitated by the nation's cadre of female community health volunteers (FCHVs) located throughout the country.

- Improved coverage of safe motherhood programmes, iron-folic acid supplementation to all pregnant women and breastfeeding mothers, deworming, maternal care and child survival interventions.

Nepal created the FCHV programme in 1988 to improve community participation and increase health service outreach. It had expanded to cover all 75 of the country's districts by 1993, but its effectiveness was hampered by frequent shortages of medical supplies, affecting volunteers' credibility. The turning point came that same year, when the national vitamin A programme was launched, with the support of the United States Agency for International Development (USAID), UNICEF, local researchers and non-governmental organizations.

This transformed the FCHVs into the most crucial component of vitamin A supplementation efforts.

By 2006, nearly 50,000 FCHVs were working throughout Nepal. In 2007, they provided vitamin A capsules to 3.5 million preschool children, maintaining coverage above 90 per cent. Beginning in 1999, deworming tablets for children aged 12 to 59 months were also distributed during the twice-yearly vitamin A supplementation.

The work of the FCHVs has expanded beyond vitamin A supplementation and deworming. These volunteers participate in community-based integrated management of childhood illnesses (diarrhoea, acute respiratory infections, measles and acute malnutrition); educate pregnant women, parents and caregivers about nutrition; distribute oral rehydration salts; provide iron and folic acid tablets to pregnant women; and spread information about nutrition, health and family planning.

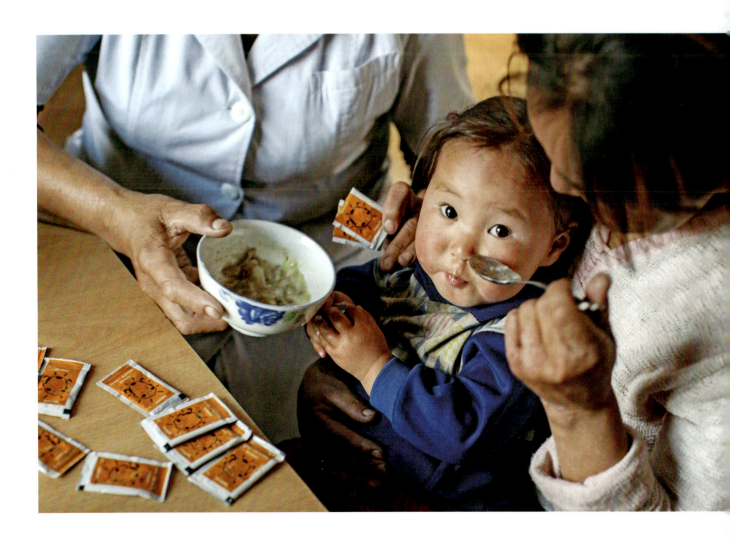

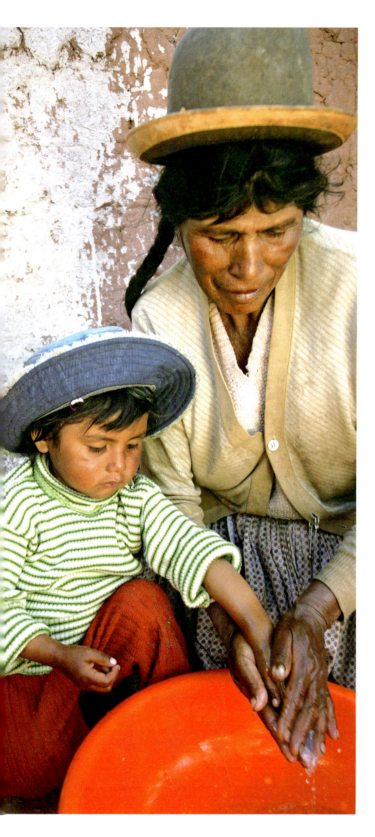

In addition, the government has worked steadily to improve coverage of key interventions. Vitamin A deficiency is believed to be largely under control, and 80 per cent of households use adequately iodized salt.[87] The proportion of children under age 5 with symptoms of pneumonia who sought treatment in a health facility increased from 18 per cent in 1996 to 50 per cent in 2011.[88] The proportion of children with diarrhoea taken to a health provider for treatment increased from 14 per cent in 1996 to 38 per cent in 2011.[89]

Although 70 per cent of infants 0–5 months are exclusively breastfed, appropriate infant and young child feeding remains a challenge. One third of infants do not begin receiving complementary foods at 6–8 months, and only 24 per cent of children aged 6–23 months are fed the recommended minimum acceptable diet with the appropriate frequency and adequate diversity.[90] The FCHVs participated in a successful pilot programme to distribute micronutrient powders for complementary feeding, and there are plans for national scale-up by 2017. The government is also looking at a social protection scheme to improve infant and young child feeding, especially among the poorest and most vulnerable people. Nepal has now developed a comprehensive national IYCF strategy to accelerate improvements in optimal infant and young child feeding and care.

Looking forward

Nepal has joined the SUN movement, and the government recently launched a multi-sectoral nutrition plan under the Prime Minister's leadership. The plan aims to address both the immediate and the underlying and basic causes of undernutrition with a package of nutrition-specific and nutrition-sensitive interventions, both based on evidence, focusing on the critical 1,000-day window including the mother's pregnancy and the child's first two years. The plan engages the National Planning Commission and five line ministries covering health, education, water and sanitation, agriculture, and local development and social protection. ■

Peru: Reaching the most disadvantaged by concentrating on equity

Between 1995 and 2005, stunting prevalence among children under 5 in Peru fluctuated but did not improve substantially. But in just a few years following the Child Malnutrition Initiative, which began in 2006, stunting fell by a third – from an estimated 30 per cent in 2004–2006 to 20 per cent in 2011.[91] Stunting prevalence among the poorest children declined from 56 per cent to 44 per cent over the same time period.[92]

Before 2005, nutrition programmes had concentrated on food assistance. But pilot programmes supported by international and non-governmental organizations began showing the effectiveness of integrated, multi-sectoral approaches in reducing stunting in rural areas. The Good Start in Life initiative, begun in 1999 and supported by UNICEF and USAID, delivered an integrated package of community-based interventions to more than 200 vulnerable communities in the Andean highlands and Amazon forest. An evaluation found that stunting among children under 3 in these communities fell from 54 per cent to 37 per cent between 2000 and 2004.[93] Similarly, CARE's REDESA (Sustainable Supply Chains for Food Security) project showed promising results in lifting families out of poverty and reducing stunting among children under 3 – from 34 per cent in 2002 to 24 per cent in 2006.[94] These pilot programmes showed that interventions can be delivered on a larger scale, with good results.

Key strategy: Raising malnutrition on the national agenda

In early 2006, international agencies and non-governmental organizations in Peru formed the Child Malnutrition Initiative with the goal of placing nutrition high on the national agenda. They advocated with policymakers to raise their awareness of the magnitude of undernutrition, its impact on national social and economic development, and the lack of progress in tackling the problem, pointing to the achievements of small-scale programmes as evidence of the potential of low-cost interventions. Before the 2006 presidential election, the Initiative lobbied candidates to sign a '5 by 5 by 5' commitment to reduce stunting in children under 5 by 5 per cent in 5 years and to lessen the inequities between urban and rural areas.

When the new government was formed later that year the fight against stunting became central to its agenda, and it has remained so. The Child Malnutrition Initiative advocated for more resources and supportive policies for child nutrition, with a focus on the most deprived households and communities. It placed special emphasis on strengthening mechanisms to identify, target, deliver and monitor efforts to reach the poorest people in rural areas.

In 2007, the government initiated the National Strategy for Poverty Reduction and Economic Opportunities (CRECER), focusing on children and pregnant women in the poorest areas. It sought to improve nutrition by strengthening multi-sectoral programmes at regional and national levels.

Several social protection and poverty reduction strategies were brought under CRECER's umbrella. The government's targeted conditional cash transfer programme, Juntos, shifted towards multi-sectoral actions to reduce child undernutrition, increase families' use of maternal and child health care services, and improve children's school attendance. The Ministry of Women and Social Development consolidated six food distribution programmes to optimize its work. A common action framework was created for the ministries of Women and Social Development, Health, Education, Agriculture, Housing and Employment, supported by sectoral budgets. Management, technical and analytical capacities were strengthened locally, regionally and nationally. Results-based financing implemented by the Ministry of Economy and Finance helped mobilize resources, improve operational efficiency and increase government accountability. Regional governments and districts adopted CRECER and took ownership of local programmes.

Over time, age-appropriate infant and young child feeding (IYCF) practices have improved *(Figure 30)*, and in 2011, rates of exclusive breastfeeding were more than twice as high among the poorest children than the richest.[95]

Key elements of Peru's success include:

- Creation of a coalition of international agencies and non-governmental organizations: The coalition advocated for commitment to reducing malnutrition.

- Capitalization on a political window of opportunity in the electoral cycle: Nutrition moved higher on the national agenda as a result.

- Strong government commitment: The issue of nutrition was placed under the direct control of the Prime Minister's office.

- Evidence from well-designed and evaluated programmes: Demonstrating the possibilities for success, these programmes fed into the design of a comprehensive, integrated national strategy, CRECER.

- Commitment to equity: This led to targeting of vulnerable groups and development of the capacity to follow up.

- Decentralization of administrative, financial and political responsibilities and adoption of a results-based budgeting mechanism: More effective financial management has improved operational efficiency.

FIGURE 30 **Peru: Infant and young child feeding practices have improved**

Infant feeding practices in Peru, by age, 1992 and 2008

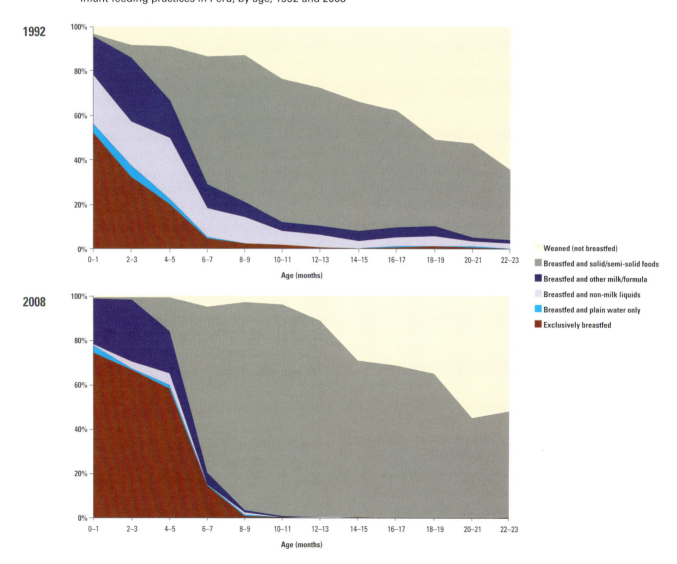

Note: See 'Interpreting IYCF area graphs' on page 104 for a description of these charts and how to read them.
Source: Peru DHS, 1992 and 2008.

Looking forward

Peru's commitment to reducing child undernutrition has been successfully translated into action. Thanks to interventions supported by CRECER, stunting has fallen substantially over a short period of time. Yet more needs to be done. More than half a million children under the age of 5 are too short for their age.[96] Inequalities have narrowed nationally, but they persist: Over the past five years, stunting rates among the poorest children have remained 10 times higher than among the richest.[97]

Peru must now turn to maintaining its commitment to scaling up nutrition and ensure the sustainability of recent successes, despite political and economic challenges. The country has underscored its commitment by joining the SUN movement and renewing its pledge to reduce the prevalence of chronic malnutrition. The newly created Ministry of Inclusion and Social Development, which leads the intersectoral coordination of nutrition, is working to further reduce inequities. ■

Rwanda: Reducing stunting through consolidated nationwide action

In 2005, more than half of Rwanda's children under 5 (nearly 800,000) were stunted. Just five years later, stunting prevalence had decreased from an estimated 52 per cent to 44 per cent.[98] This success was achieved through multi-sectoral approaches, led by the government, and the scaling up of community-based nutrition programming to all of the country's 30 districts.

Rwanda had been working to improve social services for some time. These efforts included a nearly universal community-based health insurance scheme and health financing and delivery of community-based nutrition programmes in districts since the 1990s. A boost for nutrition came when advocacy led to consolidated nationwide action. Strong evidence on the effectiveness of nutrition interventions and programme successes in parts of the country persuaded the government of the importance of investing in nutrition and demonstrated the possibility of eliminating undernutrition.

Key strategy: Transitioning a national emergency plan into a community-centred approach

In April 2009, building on the previous community-based nutrition programmes and energized by the personal interest of the nation's President, Rwanda initiated a National Emergency Plan to Eliminate Malnutrition (EPEM). This move created new momentum and led to opportunities to strengthen collaboration between sectors and support innovative programming.

The EPEM addressed both acute and chronic undernutrition, focusing first on the most vulnerable. Village-level identification and treatment of severe acute malnutrition in facilities was scaled up beginning in 2009. Around 30,000 community health workers received refresher training on how to screen, identify and refer cases for treatment.

At the same time, additional preventive measures were initiated in communities to improve household food security and care practices nationwide.

Interventions to assure sustainable household food security included expanding kitchen gardens and increasing the availability of livestock. Behaviour change interventions helped promote optimal maternal and child care and feeding practices, and growth monitoring was combined with nutrition programming in 15,000 villages. Monthly data collection and analysis at district and national levels helped to monitor progress and improve planning. It should be noted that in 2010, 85 per cent of infants aged 0–5 months were exclusively breastfed in Rwanda, and almost 80 per cent of infants 6-8 months received timely introduction to solid, semi-solid or soft foods.

Lessons learned from the EPEM were incorporated into the subsequent National Multisectoral Strategy to Eliminate Malnutrition (NmSEM) in 2010. This strategy is being implemented primarily in communities, guided by district-level multi-sectoral plans to strengthen and scale up nutrition interventions. The emphasis is on behaviour change communication to promote optimal nutrition practices during pregnancy and the first two years of the child's life.

Responsive planning and monitoring at the local level have been bolstered by improvements in information-gathering capacity. An electronic health monitoring and information system integrates nutrition data and other local information, allowing for evaluation of district-level performance. More recently, technological advances are supporting real-time collection of data on stunting – for example, rapid SMS will be used nationwide to track children's progress during their first two years.

The elements of Rwanda's approach include:

- Strong national resolve to eliminate malnutrition, by both the national government (championed by the President) and citizens.

- Rapid action to implement an emergency response followed by development of a long-term multi-sectoral strategy that incorporated lessons learned from earlier experiences.

- A community-centred approach to reducing stunting, with investment in both food security and behaviour change strategies to promote optimal nutrition practices in a sustainable manner.

- Decentralized planning, with strong monitoring and evaluation systems to improve programme performance.

Looking forward

Rwanda joined the SUN movement in 2011, signalling its ongoing commitment to addressing undernutrition. The government now develops an annual Joint Action Plan to eliminate undernutrition. Coordination mechanisms need further strengthening as the nation transitions from sector-specific to multi-sectoral planning and implementation. Rwanda is also working to maintain the quality of its interventions during the national scale-up, along with timely monitoring for continual improvement. Additional resources will be needed to invest in these efforts. In overcoming these challenges, Rwanda hopes to deliver on its vision of eliminating undernutrition across the country. ■

Democratic Republic of the Congo: Scaling up community-based management of severe acute malnutrition

In the Democratic Republic of the Congo, severe acute malnutrition affected nearly 1 million children in 2011. However, a community-based approach is dramatically increasing the number of children receiving treatment for SAM – from fewer than 46,000 in 2007 to 157,000 in 2011.[99]

Until about a decade ago, efforts to treat SAM were mostly concentrated in the conflict-affected eastern provinces and were carried out mainly by humanitarian NGOs. To harmonize interventions, the government adopted a national protocol in 2002. It required hospitalization of all children with SAM, whether or not they had medical complications. This approach proved difficult to implement, given the limited number of treatment centres and the burden of hospitalization on families.

Key strategy: Evidence-based advocacy to build broad support for action

In 2008, the country's Ministry of Health undertook to address this problem. With technical support from Valid International and other NGOs, a protocol was developed that included community-based treatment, allowing parents to treat most children at home. Initially, the protocol was implemented mainly in the eastern provinces, but the following year surveys found that acute malnutrition was even more prevalent in four central and western provinces.[100]

Survey data were key to efforts to persuade the government to address undernutrition across the whole country, as well as to make the case for more funding with donors and for more presence in the central and western regions with NGOs. The community-based protocol was revised to ensure integration of SAM treatment into primary health services and to emphasize the importance of preventive interventions such as counselling and promotion of good infant and young child feeding and hygiene practices.

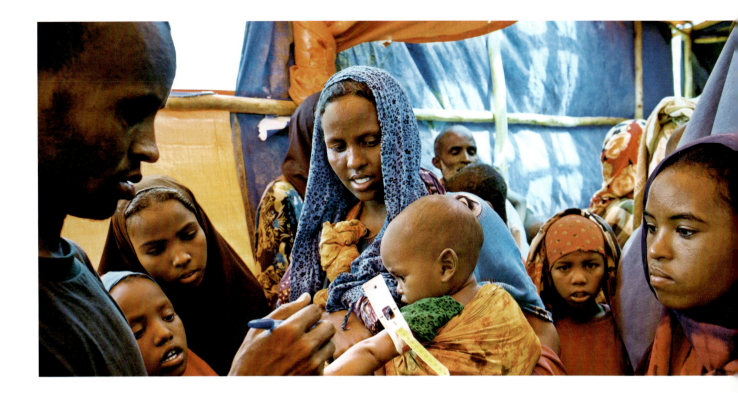

Capacity development was fostered through training sessions on emergency nutrition, the detection and management of acute malnutrition, and the 'cluster approach' to coordination and partnership. Developing the capacity of partners working at the community level and coordinating their actions helped to improve local ownership of programmes, thus solidifying efforts to implement the nutrition programme nationally.

The results were significant. Between 2007 and 2011, the number of children admitted for treatment more than tripled.[101] Treatment of SAM has been integrated into the minimum health package and in health facilities is addressed along with illnesses such as malaria, pneumonia and diarrhoea. Ready-to-use therapeutic food has been added to the Ministry of Health's list of essential drugs. Geographic coverage reportedly increased from 143 health zones in 2007 (28 per cent) to 270 in 2011 (52 per cent).[102]

Factors that contributed to these successes included:

- Development of government policy, including the change in protocol that allowed for treatment of SAM at home.

- Improved surveillance and analysis of the problem through the monitoring surveys.

- Advocacy with the government, donors and NGOs on the national nature of the problem, based on survey results.

- Effective training to build the capacity of government and NGO staff.

- NGO capacity to expand coverage where government capacity was initially limited.

- Increase of humanitarian funding for treatment of SAM between 2007 and 2011.[103]

This experience shows that emergency interventions can be a model for scaling up nutrition programmes.

Looking forward

In 2011, approximately 800,000 children suffering from SAM still lacked access to treatment.[104] One of the reasons for this limited access is that poor families have to pay out-of-pocket for health and nutrition services. In addition, about 5 million of the country's children suffer from stunting, accounting for nearly 20 per cent of the burden in West and Central Africa.[105] With the support of donors and the international community, the government is committed to scaling up SAM treatment to all health centres in every district, at a cost families can afford. ■

Sri Lanka: Reducing under-five mortality by expanding breastfeeding

Sri Lanka is a lower-middle-income country that has successfully improved child health and nutrition over the past two decades. Between 1990 and 2011, the under-five mortality rate fell from 29 to 12 deaths per 1,000 live births and the infant mortality rate fell from 24 to 11 deaths per 1,000 live births.[106] Progress has been made in breastfeeding – the exclusive breast-feeding rate among infants up to 6 months of age increased from 53 per cent in 2000 to 76 per cent in 2006–2007. The most recent estimates show that 80 per cent of babies are breastfed within the first hour after birth.[107] Yet, Sri Lanka has pockets of inequity: Undernutrition rates are higher in rural areas and in the tea-growing estates of the highlands than in other parts of the country.

Key strategy: Legislation and services to support breastfeeding mothers

Sri Lanka's achievements in improving exclusive breastfeeding rates are the result of:

- High levels of political commitment, leading to protective legislation.

- A well-developed health-care system and an enabling environment.

- A committed group of professionals and organizations that championed breastfeeding.

- A dedicated and well-trained field workforce of public health midwives reaching mothers before, during and after delivery.

- Multiple strategies for extensive awareness creation at all levels, especially among mothers' support groups.

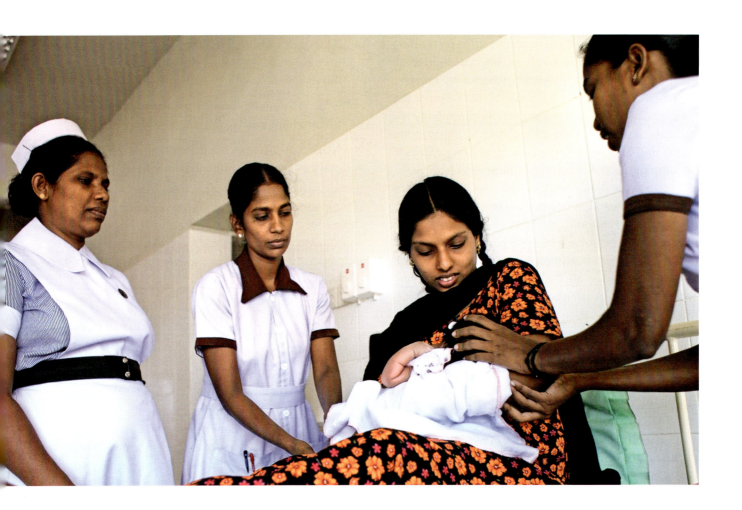

Women make up more than 30 per cent of the workforce in Sri Lanka, and the government has addressed their participation by passing maternity protection laws. In 1992, paid maternity leave in government jobs was extended from 6 weeks to 84 working days. Women in the private sector are also entitled to a 60- to 120-minute paid nursing break every nine hours during their work day for a year. In 1981, the nation was one of the first to adopt the International Code of Marketing of Breast-milk Substitutes as law, expanding it in 1993 and revising it in 2002. At the Ministry of Health's request, UNICEF provided technical support for a revised Code to address weaknesses in late 2011.

Beyond legislation, cross-sectoral programming supports outreach to mothers. A key factor in Sri Lanka's success has been the contribution of over 7,000 government-trained midwives, who are part of the public health team responsible for providing comprehensive maternal and child health care. The midwives provide post-partum care to mothers and support them in adopting appropriate breastfeeding practices – each mother receives four home visits from the midwife during the first six weeks after delivery.

Sri Lanka has developed a 40-hour training course in lactation management and delivered it to an estimated 10,000 paediatricians, obstetricians and nurses – almost the entire health workforce. Mother-baby and lactation management centres have been set up in all major hospitals to provide mothers with breast-feeding support, and print, radio and social media materials promote awareness of appropriate infant feeding practices and the benefits of breastfeeding. Studies on infant and young child feeding practices help guide programme development.

Looking forward

Sri Lanka has joined the SUN movement and is addressing undernutrition as a priority through high-level commitment and evidenced-based programming. A National Nutrition Council, established in 2011 and chaired by the President of the country, is focusing on preventing stunting and controlling malnutrition during pregnancy and in the first two years of the child's life. ■

Kyrgyzstan: Reducing iron deficiency with home fortification of food

Kyrgyzstan is one of the poorest countries in Europe and Central Asia, with approximately one in three people living in poverty. The effects of the global economic crisis, increasing food prices and political instability have had an impact on vulnerable groups, including women and children.[108]

Yet, Kyrgyzstan has become one of the first countries in the world to scale up home fortification of complementary food for children aged 6 to 23 months.

Key strategy: A successful pilot programme and nationwide education

In 1997, Kyrgyzstan's national Demographic and Health Survey showed that almost half of the nation's children under 36 months of age were anaemic, mainly due to a deficiency of iron,[109] which is crucial to a child's development, especially during the first years of life. Anaemia was a major public health challenge.

In 2007, a study found that just two months' use of micronutrient powder (MNP) reduced anaemia prevalence by 28 per cent among children 6 to 36 months old.[110] In 2009, the Ministry of Health launched a pilot MNP home fortification programme to reach children aged 6 to 23 months in Talas Province.

Single-serving MNP sachets, which could be mixed at home into solid or semi-solid complementary foods, were distributed to families by health-care providers at government clinics through a programme called Gulazyk, a Kyrgyz word referring to a dried meat product rich in nutrients and energy that was traditionally eaten by warriors or travellers to give them strength. A slogan was developed: 'Gulazyk – For the health and mind of your child'.

Each child's caregiver was given 30 MNP sachets, enough to administer one to the child roughly every other day for two months. Caregivers were instructed to make sure that all 30 sachets were given within the two months and not to administer more than one sachet per day. Community counselling was available to address problems.

At the same time, a national campaign on maternal, infant and young child nutrition was developed to educate caregivers on diet during pregnancy and the importance of exclusive breastfeeding and adequate complementary feeding. It was developed by the government with partners that included the United States Centers for Disease Control and Prevention (CDC),

UNICEF and the Swiss Red Cross. Village health volunteers educated parents on early childhood development, showing them how to promote learning and giving them a Gulazyk-branded children's book to read to their child. Media messaging promoted optimal feeding, and extensive monitoring ensured successful outcomes.

In 2008, before the MNP pilot programme was launched, a baseline survey of the nutritional status of children in Talas Province had been undertaken by UNICEF and the CDC. A follow-up survey in 2010, a year after initiation of the pilot, showed a decline in iron deficiency anaemia from 46 to 33 per cent,[111] and that 99 per cent of caretakers had heard of Gulazyk.

There were challenges – MNPs were first distributed when seasonal diarrhoea was high, and mothers associated this with the micronutrient powder. The government worked hard to show that the intervention was safe, effective and cost-efficient.

The factors that led to the success of the programme included:

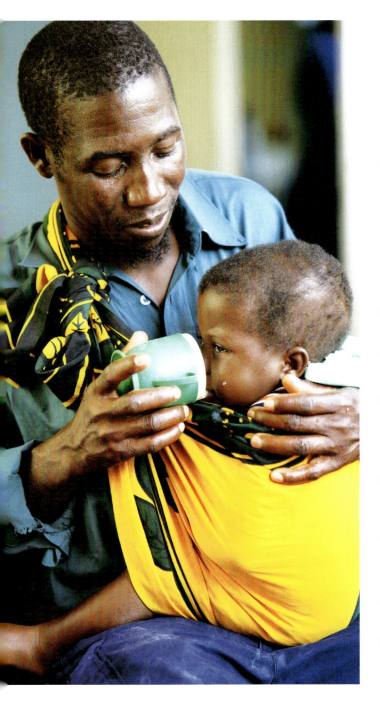

- A successful pilot programme, showing the potential of the intervention.

- An effective distribution strategy, implemented by dedicated local health-care providers.

- Communication and social mobilization at all levels, from communities to mass media, with clear arguments and messages supporting the intervention.

- Provision of learning opportunities for early childhood development, appealing to mothers, which contributed to high adherence.

- A comprehensive monitoring and evaluation system, which showed the effectiveness of MNPs and supported national scale-up.

- The support of government and other high-level decision-makers and broad partnerships.

- Involvement of a broad range of stakeholders in design, implementation and advocacy – from local nurses to professors, scientists and politicians.

Looking forward

As part of its national nutrition programme, Kyrgyzstan is now reaching 250,000 children with Gulazyk. Local production of MNPs is under consideration, and the government is working to evaluate the programme's performance and impact. The initiative has clearly shown that iron deficiency anaemia can be reduced in children aged 6 to 23 months. As the programme is scaled up nationwide, careful and continuous monitoring and evaluation are expected to ensure quality and reach, show results and maintain the support of all stakeholders. The country has joined the SUN movement and is committed to scaling up nutrition programming to benefit all of its children. ■

United Republic of Tanzania: Institutionalizing vitamin A supplementation

The United Republic of Tanzania has maintained high coverage of vitamin A supplementation (VAS) among children aged 6–59 months since twice-yearly supplementation events were introduced in 2001.[112] Between 2005 and 2011, national coverage of vitamin A supplementation has consistently exceeded 90 per cent.[113] High coverage is one of the key factors in the country's declining rate of child mortality,[114] from 126 deaths per 1,000 live births in 2000 to 68 per 1,000 in 2011.[115]

The country has maintained this coverage and in recent years has been working to strengthen national and district ownership by empowering local government authorities to take responsibility for planning and budgeting the vitamin A programme. The United Republic of Tanzania is among a group of countries taking the initiative to build national and local ownership of vitamin A programming.

Key strategy: Using Health Basket Funds to maintain coverage

Vitamin A supplements are delivered to children aged 6 to 59 months through twice-yearly events and routine health services. Until 2006, operational costs to support supplementation in each of the country's districts were funded directly by UNICEF; a more sustainable, government-led solution was thus needed. For the 2007–2008 fiscal year, funds contributed by the Canadian International Development Agency to UNICEF for the operational costs of VAS (US$ 500,000) were channelled to districts through the Health Basket Fund of the Ministry of Health and Social Welfare. This arrangement continued until fiscal year 2010–2011.

Health Basket Funds are not earmarked for specific interventions, so it was essential to ensure that districts allocated adequate resources for VAS in their annual budgets. Helen Keller International helped strengthen district capacity to plan and budget for the operational costs of distributing supplements, working through A2Z, the USAID Micronutrient and Child Blindness Project, in collaboration with the government's Tanzania Food and Nutrition Centre and UNICEF. Advocacy and capacity development events are organized during the annual planning and budgeting cycle to inform district health departments about the benefits of VAS and to strengthen planning and budgeting capacity.

A VAS sustainability assessment in 2007 had led to the creation of a simple, spreadsheet-based planning and budgeting tool, which was introduced in 2008 to help districts determine financial, human resource and supply needs. District health management teams were equipped with information, evidence and skills to defend VAS budgets to local government authorities. Advocacy was focused on district executive directors and councillors involved in decision-making. District financial allocations and VAS coverage rates were closely monitored to track the impact of all these efforts and ensure there were no negative consequences of transferring responsibility for planning and budgeting to the districts. Districts that budgeted insufficient funds or that had low VAS coverage were targeted for more intensive advocacy, including sustainability assessments and additional training.

Several factors supported the institutionalization of VAS:

- Strong partnerships were fostered among international agencies, NGOs, donors and the national government. Partners sought to find feasible solutions to promote VAS, building on knowledge generated from earlier studies.

- Sustained advocacy ensured that the benefits of VAS were understood by decision-makers and planners at national and district levels, assuring that funds were earmarked for this intervention.

- Practical steps were taken to develop capacity and create tools to empower local governments to take responsibility for district planning and budget allocation, together with close monitoring to track implementation.

- A flexible financing mechanism existed through Health Basket Funds, which offered a more sustainable source of funding.

Districts increased their allocation of Health Basket Funds for VAS more than fourfold from 2004–2005 to 2010–2011. High VAS coverage was sustained when responsibility for planning and budgeting was transferred to local government.

Looking forward

Beyond expanding coverage of vitamin A supplementation, this experience has provided an entry point to improve the planning and budgeting of other nutrition services in the United Republic of Tanzania. A new budget line for nutrition was introduced in 2012, and nutrition is now a priority in the Ministry of Finance's national planning and budgeting guidelines. District and regional teams have been oriented on how to integrate nutrition into plans and budgets in four sectors (health, agriculture, community development, and education). Public expenditure reviews on nutrition are being used to track budget allocations and expenditures on nutrition. The country joined the SUN movement in 2011, showing its willingness to make further progress on nutrition for the nation's children. ∎

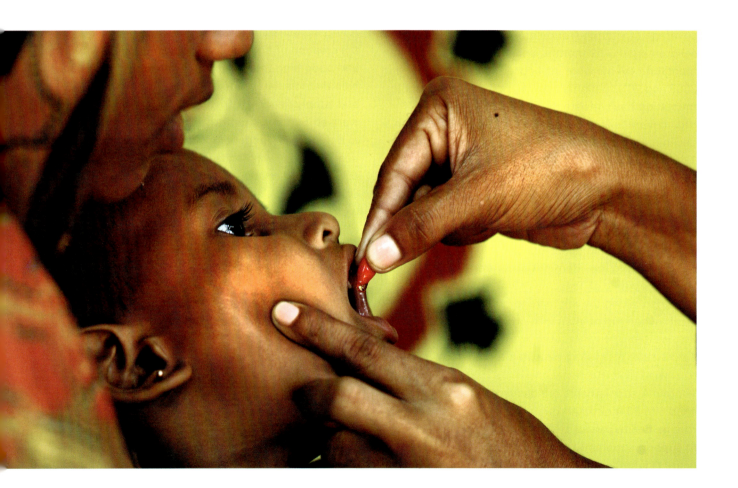

Viet Nam: Protecting breastfeeding through legislation

Viet Nam's exclusive breastfeeding rates, at about 17 per cent, have not improved since 1997;[116] they have been hindered by inadequate provisions of maternity leave and aggressive promotion of breast-milk substitutes. A 2011 study by Alive & Thrive, an initiative promoting good infant and young child feeding practices, cited returning to work as one of the main reasons mothers stopped exclusive breastfeeding. At the same time, poor regulation of marketing of breastmilk substitutes had made artificial feeding extremely popular in the Asia-Pacific region. The region accounts for 31 per cent of global retail value of baby food sales, compared with 24 per cent in Western Europe and 22 per cent in North America.[117] In response, Viet Nam's National Assembly recently enacted legislation that extends paid maternity leave and bans advertising of breastmilk substitutes for infants up to 24 months.

Key strategy: Joint advocacy by diverse partners to persuade lawmakers

The new legislation is the result of an advocacy strategy implemented by a group of partners that included the Vietnamese National Assembly's Institute of Legislative Studies, the Ministry of Health, UNICEF, the World Health Organization, Alive & Thrive and other organizations. The partners drew legislators' attention to the 1981 International Code of Marketing of Breast-milk Substitutes and subsequent World Health Assembly resolutions and the 2000 International Labour Organization Maternity Protection Convention and Recommendation. These international regulatory frameworks were used to persuade legislators of the need to protect the nutritional and breastfeeding rights of mothers and their babies. Also highlighted were the government's obligations under the Convention on the Rights of the Child, which addresses breastfeeding specifically in article 24.

Information on the proposed legislation was provided to the 200 members of the National Assembly and to policy advisers from Provincial Parliament Offices during consultative meetings held at regional and provincial levels. Participants discussed the scientific evidence on breastfeeding, international standards and the socio-economic challenges to meeting the standards.

They learned that breastmilk substitutes are vulnerable to mixing mistakes, manufacturing errors and contamination, which contribute to increases in disease and child death.

Advocacy efforts paid off. On 21 June 2012, the National Assembly passed a Law on Advertisement banning promotion of breastmilk substitutes for children up to the age of 24 months. A provision in the Labour Code extending paid maternity leave from four to six months also passed by an overwhelming majority. Both these provisions were passed with more than 90 per cent of the votes.

The combination of strategies that helped Viet Nam achieve these results included:

- Identification of key operational partners and of their comparative advantage in influencing policy dialogue and evidence generation.

- Use of stakeholder mapping to identify key counterparts: the Ministry of Health; the Ministry of Labour, Invalids and Social Affairs; the Women's Union; the General Confederation of Labour; and the Institute of Legislative Studies.

- Monitoring of progress and updates from counterparts, including daily updates prior to approval of the law, which helped spur timely action.

- Careful preparation of evidence-based advocacy materials illustrating the problem; explaining the harmful health, social and economic impact for individuals, families, communities and the nation as a whole; and providing information on regulatory solutions within the context of internationally agreed instruments.

- Face-to-face advocacy with counterparts, providing consistent messages, evidence, facts and statistics to support the course of action being recommended.

The process was arduous at times. Some National Assembly members and other stakeholders became hesitant to expand the advertising ban when interest groups raised concerns about violation of international trade laws. The partners responded with proof that the measures were perfectly compatible with world trade rules. They also maintained that adoption of the proposed measures would improve the country's efforts to fulfil its obligations under the Convention on the Rights of the Child. In addition, they provided evidence from a monitoring exercise that revealed the harmful marketing practices that were taking place, the impact on child development and the extent to which the country was lagging behind the rest of the world in terms of protection, promotion and support of breastfeeding.

Another barrier was the assumption that employers and even female workers themselves did not want extended maternity leave. This was addressed through a survey by the General Confederation of Labour, which found that 80 per cent of employers and nearly 90 per cent of female workers supported six months of paid maternity leave. The government confirmed that funds were sufficient to cover the cost. As an added persuasion, estimates were presented suggesting that the effect of improved breastfeeding practices on children's health in later life could help Viet Nam save millions of dollars in long-term health-care costs.

Looking forward

The next steps include monitoring enforcement of this new legislation and educating mothers and communities on the importance of breastfeeding their babies, particularly exclusive breastfeeding for the first six months. The partners will support the Government of Viet Nam in disseminating information, developing the capacities of key stakeholders such as health workers and ensuring that all primary-health-care facilities provide skilled counselling and support for breastfeeding so that all mothers have access to these services close to their homes. ■

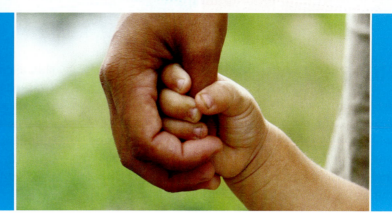

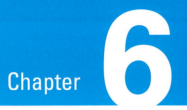

Chapter 6

NEW DEVELOPMENTS IN GLOBAL PARTNERSHIPS

Improving nutrition, particularly of children and women, is increasingly recognized as imperative for reducing poverty, promoting sustainable social and economic development and narrowing inequities. The existence of solutions and the formation of new partnerships committed to taking action have created an unprecedented opportunity to address child undernutrition through country-led, cross-sectoral actions based on evidence. This report does not review all of these partnerships, but rather highlights two initiatives in which UNICEF plays a major role.

Scaling Up Nutrition

Launched in 2010, the SUN movement is catalysing action to build national commitment to accelerate progress in reducing undernutrition and stunting. It works through implementation of evidence-based nutrition interventions and integration of nutrition goals across diverse sectors – health, social protection, poverty alleviation, national development and agriculture – focusing on the window of opportunity of the 1,000 days covering pregnancy and the child's first two years.

Globally, more than 30 countries have joined the SUN movement and are working with multiple stakeholders to scale up their nutrition programmes, supported by donor countries, United Nations organizations, civil society and the private sector. Working together, these stakeholders support country-led efforts to scale up nutrition, increasing access to resources, both financial and technical, to improve coordination of nutrition-specific interventions and

nutrition-sensitive approaches. SUN focuses on both the short term (recognizing nutrition's crucial role in improving maternal and child health) and the long term (building the foundation for a healthy, more prosperous future and resilience in times of crisis).

The SUN movement Lead Group was established in 2012 by the United Nations Secretary-General to improve coherence, provide strategic oversight, improve resource mobilization and ensure collective accountability. Members of the Lead Group are high-level leaders who represent the array of partners engaged in SUN, including heads of state, donors, civil society, business and the United Nations system. In September 2012, the Lead Group agreed to a new strategy with specific, measurable targets for the next two to three years. More work is needed to encourage countries to join SUN – just 5 of the 10 countries with the highest burden of stunting have joined the movement.

REACH

A key partner in SUN is REACH – Renewed Efforts Against Child Hunger and Undernutrition – under which the World Food Programme, UNICEF, the Food and Agriculture Organization of the United Nations and the World Health Organization have made commitments. REACH helps to coordinate multiple agencies and governments, including ministries of health, agriculture, education and finance, as they design and implement national child undernutrition policies and programmes.

REACH is increasing the emphasis on strengthening nutrition management and governance while also supporting multi-sectoral nutrition actions, including nutrition-sensitive programmatic approaches. This shift aligns with the SUN movement, which has stressed the need for nutrition-sensitive development. Donors and other partners consider REACH a valuable capacity-development and coordination mechanism for mainstreaming nutrition management and governance, as well as a key vehicle for supporting SUN in countries.

REACH is currently operational in 13 countries: Bangladesh, Ethiopia, Ghana, the Lao People's Democratic Republic, Mali, Mauritania, Mozambique, Nepal, Niger, Rwanda, Sierra Leone, Uganda and the United Republic of Tanzania. REACH is working in synergy with SUN, helping to plan implementation of Sierra Leone's food and nutrition policy, for example, and acting as a catalyst in establishing a civil society alliance for SUN in Bangladesh.

BOX 5 **Millennium Development Goals Achievement Fund –
Joint programming for children, food security and nutrition**

The MDG Achievement Fund (MDG-F or MDG-Fund) was established in 2007 following an agreement between the Government of Spain and the United Nations system. The aim was to accelerate progress towards achievement of the MDGs, primarily by supporting 130 joint programmes in 50 countries in thematic areas corresponding to the goals. A central tenet of the MDG-Fund's programmes is their 'jointness'– bringing together multiple United Nations agencies to 'deliver as one' at the country level, in keeping with the common United Nations Development Assistance Framework.

UNICEF is the lead convenor agency for the Children, Food Security and Nutrition thematic area, covering 24 joint programmes. Each of these has tried to spur innovation by capitalizing on the strengths and expertise of the individual partners and encouraging all to focus on achieving strong and equitable results.

For example, in Timor-Leste, multiple United Nations agencies and national partners are working to improve complementary feeding practices through numerous activities. These include cultivating home gardens and aquaculture to improve access to diverse, locally available foods and generate income; holding cooking demonstrations to educate mothers about how to prepare safe, nutritious foods; and working with mother support groups to improve knowledge of safe infant and young child feeding practices.

The joint programme in Mauritania is working to strengthen the capacity of government officials and other stakeholders to coordinate implementation of multi-sectoral nutrition and food security policies. The programme was designed following a joint analysis conducted by REACH and its partners, benefiting from the country's previous experience in joint programming. An innovative aspect of this programme is the establishment of flexible operational coordination mechanisms at national, regional and local levels. At the local level, decentralized implementation has allowed for experimentation with different coordination mechanisms. Nutrition and food security task teams collaborate with communities to coordinate a community-owned response to undernutrition. Early results suggest that these mechanisms have improved the effectiveness of the joint programmes and encouraged local ownership. They have also provided a platform to respond flexibly to local conditions.

The work of all joint programmes is aligned with national priorities and supported by inclusive partnerships, helping to ensure programme relevance and sustainability.

Chapter 7

THE WAY FORWARD

Over the past few years, national and global interest in nutrition has increased dramatically. There are a number of reasons for this new interest.

Recurrent food shortages, rising food prices and humanitarian crises in some regions have garnered global attention. The debate on climate change and the focus on building resilience in communities under stress have also focused attention on nutrition. At the other end of the spectrum, the rising numbers of people who struggle with overweight and obesity have become more glaring.

More persuasive evidence has become available on the harmful consequences of micronutrient deficiencies and the positive impact of exclusive breastfeeding and adequate complementary feeding for adult life and the next generation. At the same time, evidence has improved on the effectiveness of programme approaches to treat conditions such as severe acute malnutrition using ready-to-use therapeutic foods and iron and folic acid deficiency using wheat flour fortification – as well as on the feasibility of implementing these programmes at scale.

Scientific knowledge and understanding have also improved regarding the linkages between stunting and rapid and disproportionate weight gain in early childhood. This has resulted in a shift in response. Previously the focus was on efforts to reduce the prevalence of underweight among children under the age of 5, an indicator of MDG 1. Now it is shifting towards prevention of stunting during the period from pregnancy up to 2 years of age.

The improved scientific evidence on the impact of interventions has enhanced advocacy to position nutrition as a sound investment for poverty reduction and social and economic development.

A unified international nutrition community has been using the Scaling Up Nutrition movement to successfully advocate for reduction of stunting, acute malnutrition and micronutrient deficiencies. This message has been heard and echoed by other initiatives and channels, including the Secretary-General's Zero Hunger Challenge, the 1,000 Days initiative and the Copenhagen Consensus 2012 Expert Panel's findings that malnourishment should be the top priority for policymakers and philanthropists. The G8 has also included action to address stunting and other forms of undernutrition in its agenda.

As of the end of 2012, the SUN message had led more than 30 countries in Africa, Asia and Latin America to scale up their nutrition programmes, supported by a wide range of organizations and, in many cases, by the donor community. This is probably the clearest indication of the growing interest in tackling stunting and other forms of undernutrition. It is crucial to maintain this momentum and to further increase the level of interest and motivation.

How can this be done? By showing that success in the foreseeable future is not only possible, but realistically achievable. The 2009 *Tracking Progress on Child and Maternal Nutrition* report showed that there was scientific evidence supporting a set of interventions to improve nutritional status. This report goes a step further, showing that programmatic approaches and the experience necessary to implement these interventions at scale exist, and that the nutritional status of populations can improve significantly as a result.

A number of common determinants are at the basis of the successful implementation of the examples described in Chapter 5. These include the political commitment to reduce stunting and other forms of undernutrition; the design and implementation of comprehensive and effective national policy and programmes based on sound situation analysis; the presence of trained and skilled community workers collaborating with communities; effective communication and advocacy; and multi-sectoral delivery of services.

These and other positive experiences must be consistently and constantly used to advocate with policymakers and decision-makers, especially those who are not familiar with nutrition and its importance for health and development. Advocacy efforts have proved effective in recent years, but more work is needed to sustain the interest and motivation of governments, particularly to maintain budgetary commitments and expansion of programmes. Global initiatives should play a major role in this effort to keep nutrition in the spotlight.

An expanded range of interventions is needed in many countries to address stunting and other nutrition indicators. Maternal nutrition has a large impact on infant nutritional status, and not enough interventions to improve maternal nutrition are being implemented at scale across countries. Many countries have an official iron-folic acid supplementation programme for pregnant women, but in most cases its implementation is not optimal. Other proven options are not being used to the fullest extent, such as multi-micronutrient supplements, improving nutrient intake using locally available foods, providing food supplements where appropriate, and deworming.

Programmes to improve complementary feeding for children aged 6 to 24 months also require expansion. The same is true of efforts to improve nutritional status among adolescent girls. Adolescence presents an opportune and receptive time to promote healthy nutrition behaviours, and this opportunity must be harnessed.

Continued research is needed to strengthen the knowledge of the causes and consequences of stunting and other forms of undernutrition. The intergenerational impact of undernutrition, and the relationship between the timing of deficiencies during pregnancy and developmental impact after birth, and between early growth retardation and overweight, are only beginning to be understood. Applied research is also required to improve an understanding of effective programme approaches and strategies to improve caring practices, reduce child overweight through stunting prevention and improve both distribution and use of food and micronutrient supplements. Lipid-based supplements have been shown to reduce stunting and improve child development, but more evidence would strengthen understanding of their impact and possible use in various target groups, such as pregnant women, and help in the design of programme strategies to reach them.

Stunting and other forms of undernutrition are also linked to health, food availability, water and sanitation, cultural practices and social and political factors. But evidence on how improving these factors affects nutritional status is still limited. Few programmes aiming to improve these factors have the co-objective of improving nutrition of women and children, so nutritional status is rarely used as an indicator to gauge their success. As a result, information on cost-effectiveness is lacking.

This report notes the need for household food security to attain optimal nutrition, but the limited evidence base on the impact of agricultural interventions on child nutrition highlights the need for more work in this area. Similarly, the impact of social safety net programmes needs further documentation to improve the effectiveness of this intervention. These issues are of special importance in countries that experience regular food shortages and need to build resilience to such shocks to prevent the tragedies that require large numbers of children to be treated for severe acute malnutrition.

Now that many countries are scaling up nutrition programmes, it is important to ensure optimal use of resources and achieve results rapidly. If programmes are not making the necessary progress, strategies need to be adapted quickly. This requires a monitoring system to assess whether bottlenecks impeding programme effectiveness are effectively addressed and the collection of information in real time rather than reliance on large-scale household survey data, which are normally collected intermittently.

Wider use of innovative technology has the potential to transform programme coverage and effectiveness. In some countries the use of mobile phones for rapid messaging has enhanced programmes in terms of supply availability, service uptake, community engagement and quality of monitoring. Much broader application is possible. There are exciting possibilities to be explored, particularly when they are paired with interventions by community workers.

The evidence demonstrating the impact of stunting and other forms of undernutrition on survival, individual and national development, and long-term health is irrefutable.

As the world looks to the post-2015 development agenda, it is clear that prevention and treatment of undernutrition must be at its core. The evidence outlined in this report, the momentum around tackling the problem, the successes already achieved and the impact on equitable and sustainable poverty reduction show that improving child and maternal nutrition is both achievable and imperative for global progress.

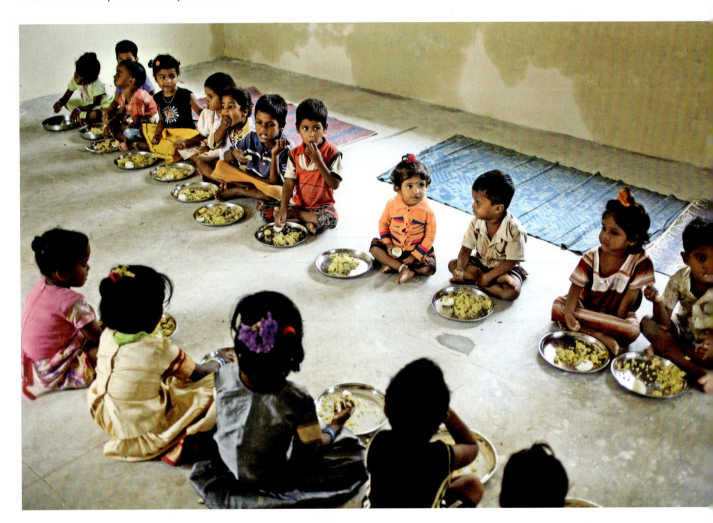

REFERENCES

CHAPTER 2

1 *Biological programming* refers to the process by which exposure to a stimulus or insult during a critical period of development can change the predisposition to developing disease, with long-term consequences.

2 Victora, Cesar G., et al., 'Worldwide Timing of Growth Faltering: Revisiting implications for interventions', *Pediatrics*, vol. 125, no. 3, 1 February 2010, p. e473.

3 Walker, Susan P., et al., 'Inequality in Early Childhood: Risk and protective factors for early child development', *Lancet*, vol. 378, no. 9799, 8 October 2011, pp. 1328, 1334.

4 Özaltin, Emre, Kenneth Hill and S. V. Subramanian, 'Association of maternal stature with offspring mortality, underweight, and stunting in low- to middle-income countries'. *JAMA*, vol. 303, no. 15, 21 April 2010, pp. 1507–1516.

5 Lawn, Joy E., Simon Cousens and Jelka Zupan, '4 Million Neonatal Deaths: When? Where? Why?', *Lancet*, vol. 365, no. 9462, 5 March 2005, p. 347.

6 UNICEF Global Databases, 2012.

7 Black, Robert E., et al., 'Maternal and Child Undernutrition: Global and regional exposures and health consequences', *Lancet*, vol. 371, no. 9608, 19 January 2008, pp. 243–260. See especially Table 2.

8 Victora, Cesar G., et al., 'Maternal and Child Undernutrition: Consequences for adult health and human capital', *Lancet*, vol. 371, no. 9609, 26 January 2008, p. 340; Almond, Douglas, and Janet Currie, 'Human Capital Development before Age Five', *Handbook of Labor Economics*, vol. 4B, 2011, pp. 1315–1486; Martorell, Reynaldo, et al., 'The Nutrition Intervention Improved Adult Human Capital and Economic Productivity', *Journal of Nutrition*, vol. 140, no. 2, February 2010, pp. 411–414.

9 Dewey, Kathryn G., and K. Begum, 'Long-term Consequences of Stunting in Early Life', *Maternal and Child Nutrition*, vol. 7, October 2011, pp. 5–18; Grantham-McGregor, S., et al., 'Developmental Potential in the First 5 Years for Children in Developing Countries', *Lancet*, vol. 369, no. 9555, 6 January 2007, p. 65.

10 Martorell, Reynaldo, et al., 'Weight Gain in the First Two Years of Life Is an Important Predictor of Schooling Outcomes in Pooled Analyses from Five Birth Cohorts from Low- and Middle-Income Countries', *Journal of Nutrition*, vol. 140, no. 2, February 2010, pp. 348–354.

11 Grantham-McGregor, S., et al., 'Developmental Potential in the First 5 Years for Children in Developing Countries', *Lancet*, vol. 369, no. 9555, 6 January 2007, p. 67.

12 Cusick, Sarah E., and Michael K. Georgieff, 'Nutrient Supplementation and Neurodevelopment: Timing Is the Key', *Archives of Pediatrics and Adolescent Medicine*, vol. 166, no. 5, May 2012, pp. 481–482.

13 Martorell, Reynaldo, et al., 'Weight Gain in the First Two Years of Life Is an Important Predictor of Schooling Outcomes in Pooled Analyses from Five Birth Cohorts from Low- and Middle-Income Countries', pp. 348–354.

14 Lien, Nguyen M., Knarig K. Meyer and Myron Winick, 'Early Malnutrition and "Late" Adoption: A study of their effects on the development of Korean orphans adopted into American families', *American Journal of Clinical Nutrition*, vol. 30, no. 10, October 1977, pp. 1738–1739.

15 Stoch, Mavis B., and P. M. Smythe, '15-year Developmental Study on Effects of Severe Undernutrition During Infancy on Subsequent Physical Growth and Intellectual Functioning', *Archives of Disease in Childhood*, vol. 51, no. 327, 1976, pp. 332–333.

16 Uauy, Ricardo, Juliana Kain and Camila Corvalan, 'How Can the Developmental Origin of Health and Disease [DOHaD] Hypothesis Contribute to Improving Health in Developing Countries?' *American Journal of Clinical Nutrition*, vol. 94, no. 6 (Suppl.), 4 May 2011, p. 1759S; Norris, Shane, et al., 'Size at Birth, Weight Gain in Infancy and Childhood, and Adult Diabetes Risk in Five Low and Middle Income Country Birth Cohorts', *Diabetes Care*, vol. 35, no. 1,

18 November 2011, pp. 72–79; Barker, David J. P., 'Maternal Nutrition, Fetal Nutrition, and Disease in Later Life', *Nutrition*, vol. 13, no. 9, September 1997, pp. 807–813.

17 Wells, Jonathan C. K., et al., 'Associations of Intrauterine and Postnatal Weight and Length Gains with Adolescent Body Composition: Prospective birth cohort study from Brazil', *Journal of Adolescent Health*, vol. 51, no. 6, December 2012, pp. S58–S64; Kuzawa, Christopher W., et al., 'Birth Weight, Postnatal Weight Gain, and Adult Body Composition in Five Low and Middle Income Countries', *American Journal of Human Biology*, vol. 24, no. 1, January–February 2012, p. S62.

18 Black et al., 'Maternal and Child Undernutrition', pp. 243–260.

CHAPTER 3

19 The values of the anthropometric indicators were calculated using the WHO standard growth reference. The sources of the data are nationally representative household surveys, such as UNICEF-supported Multiple Indicator Cluster Surveys (MICS), USAID-supported Demographic and Health Surveys (DHS) and other national surveys.

20 Global and regional estimates in this chapter reflect those consistent with the UNICEF, WHO, World Bank Joint Child Malnutrition Estimates from analysis of the Joint Global Nutrition database from 1990 to 2011. The data presented here supersede relevant historical data published by UNICEF and WHO. Further details of the harmonized methodology are available at <www.childinfo.org/malnutrition.html>.

21 UNICEF Global Nutrition Database, 2012.

CHAPTER 4

22 Walker, Susan P., et al., 'Inequality in Early Childhood: Risk and protective factors for early child development', *Lancet*, vol. 378, no. 9799, 8 October 2011, pp. 1325–1338.

23 Fall, Caroline H. D., et al., 'Multiple Micronutrient Supplementation During Pregnancy in Low-income Countries: A meta-analysis of effects on birth size and length of gestation', supplement, *Food and Nutrition Bulletin*, vol. 30, no. S 4, 2009, pp. 533–546.

24 Imdad, Aamer, and Zulfiqar A. Bhutta, 'Maternal Nutrition and Birth Outcomes: Effect of balanced protein–energy supplementation', *Paediatric and Perinatal Epidemiology*, vol. 26, no. s1, July 2012, pp. 178–190.

25 Chaparro, Camila M., and Kathryn G. Dewey, 'Use of Lipid-based Nutrient Supplements (LNS) to Improve the Nutrient Adequacy of General Food Distribution Rations for Vulnerable Sub-groups in Emergency Settings', *Maternal and Child Nutrition*, vol. 6, January 2010, pp. 1–69.

26 UNICEF Global Databases, 2012.

27 Jones, Gareth, et al., 'How Many Child Deaths Can We Prevent This Year?', *Lancet*, vol. 362, no. 9377, 5 July 2003, pp. 65–71.

28 Kramer, Michael S., et al. 'Breastfeeding and Child Cognitive Development: New evidence from a large randomized trial', *Archives of General Psychiatry*, vol. 65, no. 5, May 2008, p. 578.

29 Fall, Caroline H. D., et al., 'Infant-feeding Patterns and Cardiovascular Risk Factors in Young Adulthood: Data from five cohorts in low- and middle-income countries', *International Journal of Epidemiology*, vol. 40, no. 1, February 2011, pp. 47–62.

30 United Nations Children's Fund, *Infant and Young Child Feeding Programming Status: Results of 2010–2011 assessment of key actions for comprehensive infant and young child feeding programmes in 65 countries*, UNICEF, New York, April 2012.

31 Mullany, Luke., et al., 'Breastfeeding Patterns, Time to Initiation and Mortality Risk among Newborns in Southern Nepal', *Journal of Nutrition*, vol. 138, no. 3, March 2008, pp. 599–603; Edmond, Karen M., et al., 'Delayed Breastfeeding Initiation Increases Risk of Neonatal Mortality, *Pediatrics*, vol. 117, no. 3, 1 March 2006, pp. e380–e386.

32 UNICEF Global Nutrition Database, 2012.

33 Black et al., 'Maternal and Child Undernutrition', pp. 243–260.

34 Ibid.

35 Dewey, Kathryn G., et al., 'Effects of Age of Introduction of Complementary Foods on Iron Status of Breast-fed Infants in Honduras', *American Journal of Clinical Nutrition*, vol. 67, no. 5, May 1998, pp. 878–884; Arpadi, Stephen, et al., 'Growth Faltering due to Breastfeeding Cessation in Uninfected Children Born to HIV-infected Mothers in Zambia', August 2009, pp. 344–353.

36 UNICEF Global Nutrition Database, 2012.

37 UNICEF Global Nutrition Database, 2012, subset analysis of 50 countries with available trend data.

38 Bhutta Zulfiqar A., et al., 'What Works? Interventions for maternal and child undernutrition and survival', *Lancet*, vol. 371, no. 9610, 2 February 2008, pp. 417–440.

39 Dewey, Kathryn G., and Seth Adu-Afarwuah, 'Systematic Review of the Efficacy and Effectiveness of Complementary Feeding Interventions in Developing Countries', *Maternal and Child Nutrition*, vol. 4, 14 February 2008, pp. 24–85; Avula, Rasmi, et al., 'Enhancements to Nutrition Program in Indian Integrated Child Development Services Increased Growth and Energy Intake of Children', *Journal of Nutrition*, vol.141, no. 4, 1 April 2011, pp. 680–684.

40 United Nations Children's Fund, *Programming Guide, Infant and Young Child Feeding*, UNICEF, New York, June 2012.

41 Dewey, Kathryn G., 'Complementary Feeding', in *Encyclopedia of Human Nutrition*, edited by B. Caballero, L. Allen and A. Prentice, Elsevier Ltd., Amsterdam, 2005, pp. 465–470.

42 Pan American Health Organization/World Health Organization, 'Guiding Principles for Complementary Feeding of the Breastfed Child', PAHO/WHO, Washington, D.C., 2003; United Nations Children's Fund, 'Programming Guide, Infant and Young Child Feeding', UNICEF, New York, June 2012.

43 World Health Organization, 'Global Prevalence of Vitamin A Deficiency in Populations at Risk: WHO global database on vitamin A deficiency', WHO, Geneva, 2009.

44 Benoist, Bruno de, et al., 'Worldwide Prevalence of Anaemia 1993–2005: WHO global database on anaemia', WHO, Geneva, 2008.

45 Of the 18 profiled countries with available data since 2005, the percentage of women reporting using iron-folic acid for more than 90 days was less than 50 per cent in 17 countries.

46 UNICEF Global Databases, 2012, based on 54 countries reporting national estimates of household salt iodization of at least 15ppm, 2007 – 2011.

47 Dewey, Kathryn G., Zhenyu Yang and Erick Boy, 'Systematic Review and Meta-analysis of Home Fortification of Complementary Foods', *Maternal and Child Nutrition*, vol. 5, no. 4, October 2009, pp. 283–321.

48 United Nations Children's Fund and U.S. Centers for Disease Control and Prevention, *Global Assessment of Home Fortification Interventions, 2011*, Home Fortification Technical Advisory Group, Geneva, 2012.

49 Flour Fortification Initiative, <www.ffinetwork.org/global_progress/index.php>, accessed 8 January 2012.

50 Black et al., 'Maternal and Child Undernutrition', pp. 243–260.

51 Richard, Stephanie A., et al., 'Wasting Is Associated with Stunting in Early Childhood', *Journal of Nutrition*, vol. 142, no. 7, 1 July 2012, pp. 1291–1296.

52 World Health Organization/World Food Programme/United Nations System Standing Committee on Nutrition/United Nations Children's Fund, *Community-Based Management of Severe Acute Malnutrition: A joint statement by the World Health Organization, the World Food Programme, the United Nations System Standing Committee on Nutrition and the United Nations Children's Fund*, May 2007.

53 The Sphere Project, *Humanitarian Charter and Minimum Standards in Humanitarian Response*, Belmont Press, Northampton, UK, 2011.

54 UNICEF Nutrition Section, Global Severe Acute Malnutrition Update, 2012.

55 Humphrey, Jean H., 'Child Undernutrition, Tropical Enteropathy, Toilets, and Handwashing, *Lancet*, vol. 374, 19 September 2009, pp. 1032–1035; Dangour, A. D., et al., Interventions to Improve Water Quality and Supply, Sanitation and Hygiene Practices, and Their Effects on the Nutritional Status of Children (Protocol), *The Cochrane Library* 2011, Issue 10.

56 Guerrant, Richard L., et al., 'Malnutrition as an Enteric Infectious Disease with Long-term Effects on Child Development', Article first published online: 22 August 2008. DOI: 10.1111/j.1753-4887.2008.00082.x.

57 International Food Policy Research Institute, 'Leveraging Agriculture for Improving Nutrition and Health', IFPRI, New Delhi, 2011; Herforth, Anna, 'Synthesis of Guiding Principles on Agriculture Programming for Nutrition', Draft, September 2012, Food and Agriculture Organization of the United Nations, Rome; Hoddinott, John, 'Agriculture, Health, and Nutrition: Toward conceptualizing the linkages,' paper presented at the 2020 Conference, New Delhi, India, 10–12 February 2011; Hawkes, Corrina, R. Turner and J. Waage, 'Current and Planned Research on Agriculture for Improved Nutrition: A mapping and a gap analysis', Department for International Development, London, August 2012.

58 Girard, Amy Webb, et al., 'The Effects of Household Food Production Strategies on the Health and Nutrition Outcomes of Women and Young Children: A systematic review', *Paediatric and Perinatal Epidemiology*, vol. 26, no. s1, July 2012, pp. 205–222.

59 Independent Evaluation Group (IEG), 'What Can We Learn from Nutrition Impact Evaluations?: Lessons from a review of interventions to reduce child malnutrition in developing countries', World Bank Publications, Washington, D.C., July 2010.

60 Independent Evaluation Group, ibid.

CHAPTER 5

61 These success stories draw on internal documents, government documents and expert opinion provided by UNICEF Country Offices. Additional sources include:

Ethiopia: Rajkumar, Andrew S., Christopher Gaukler and Jessica Tilahun, 'Combating Malnutrition in Ethiopia: An evidence-based approach for sustained results', Africa Human Development Series, World Bank, Washington, D.C., 2012; and Gilligan, Daniel O., et al., 'The Impact of Ethiopia Productive Safety Net Programme and its Linkages', Mimeo, International Food Policy Research Institute, Washington, D.C., December 2008.

Nepal: United States Agency for International Development and Government of Nepal, 'An Analytical Report on National Survey of Female Community Health Volunteers of Nepal', USAID and Government of Nepal, Kathmandu, 2007; United States Agency for International Development, 'Vitamin A Supplements for Children', Nepal Family Health Program, Technical Brief no. 2, USAID, Washington, D.C., 2007; and Thapa, Shyam, Minja Kim Choe and Robert D. Retherford, 'Effects of Vitamin A Supplementation on Child Mortality: Evidence from Nepal's 2001 Demographic and Health Survey', *Tropical Medicine & International Health*, vol. 10, no. 8, August 2005, pp. 782–789.

Peru: Acosta, Andrés Mejía, 'Analysing Success in the Fight against Malnutrition in Peru', IDS Working Papers, vol. 2011, no. 367, May 2011, pp. 2–49; and Garret, James, Lucy Basset and Alessandra Marini, 'Designing CCT Programs to Improve Nutrition Impact: Principles, Evidences and Examples', Hunger-Free Latin America and the Caribbean Initiative Working Paper, Food and Agriculture Organization, Santiago, Chile, 2009.

Sri Lanka: United Nations Children's Fund, *Infant and Young Child Feeding Programme Review*, UNICEF, New York, June 2009.

Krygyzstan: Ministry of Health of the Kyrgyz Republic, U.S. Centers for Disease Control and Prevention and United Nations Children's Fund, 'Assessment of the Nutritional Status of Children 6–24 Months of Age and Their Mothers: Rural Talas Oblast, Kyrgyzstan, 2008', UNICEF, Bishkek, 2010; and World Bank, 'Kyrgyz Republic Partnership: Program snapshot', World Bank, Washington, D.C., October 2012.

The United Republic of Tanzania: A2Z Project and United States Agency for International Development, 'Assessment of the Sustainability of the Tanzania National Vitamin A Supplementation Program', A2Z, Washington, D.C., 2008; and Helen Keller International and CIDA Vitamin A Program, 'A Review of Comprehensive Council Health Plans 2010/2011', 2012.

Viet Nam: Alive & Thrive, 'Maternity Leave Policy in Viet Nam: Summary report', Alive & Thrive, Ha Noi, Viet Nam, July 2012.

62 United Nations Inter-agency Group for Child Mortality Estimation, 2012.

63 Demographic and Health Surveys, 2000 and 2011.

64 UNICEF Global Databases, 2012.

65 World Bank data, 2012.

66 Rajkumar, Andrew S., Christopher Gaukler and Jessica Tilahun, 'Combating Malnutrition in Ethiopia: An evidence-based approach for sustained results', Africa Human Development Series, World Bank, Washington, D.C., 2012.

67 Berhane, Guush, et al., 'The Impact of Ethiopia's Productive Safety Nets and Household Asset Building Programme: 2006–2010', International Food Policy Research Institute, Washington, D.C., December 2011; and Gilligan, Daniel O., et al., 'The Impact of Ethiopia Productive Safety Net Programme and Its Linkages', Mimeo, International Food Policy Research Institute, Washington, D.C., December 2008.

68 Data provided by UNICEF Ethiopia, 2012.

69 The Last Ten Kilometres Project, 'Changes in Maternal, Newborn and Child Health in 115 Rural *Woredas* of Amhara, Oromia, SNNP, and Tigray Regions of Ethiopia: 2008–2010 – Findings from the L10K baseline and midterm surveys', JSI Research & Training Institute, Inc., Addis Ababa, July 2012.

70 Coordination Nationale de la Sécurité Alimentaire, 'Rapid Post-Earthquake Emergency Food Security Assessment', CNSA, Port-au-Prince, March 2010.

71 Ministère de la Santé Publique et de la Population 'Enquête nutritionelle anthropométrique et de mortalité retrospective chez les enfants de 6 à 59 mois dans les zones affectées par le seisme du 12 janvier 2010', Ministère de la Santé Publique et de la Population, Port-au-Prince, 2010.

72 World Food Programme, 'Haiti: One year after the 12 January earthquake' (communication fact sheet), 2011; and Family Early Warning Systems Network, 'Haiti Food Security Outlook', United States Agency for International Development, Washington, D.C., January 2011.

73 CNSA/MARNDR Haiti, 'Résultats de l'enquête la sécurité alimentaire EFSA II1', Famine and Early Warning Systems Network, September 2010.

74 Data provided by UNICEF Haiti, 2013.

75 Cayemittes, Michel, et al., 'Enquête mortalité, morbidité et utilisation des services EMMUS-IV: Haïti – 2005–2006', Ministère de la Santé Publique et de la Population, Institut Haïtien de l'Enfance and Macro International, Calverton, MD, January 2007.

76 Ministère de la Santé Publique et de la Population, UNICEF and World Food Programme, *Rapport de l'enquête nutritionnelle nationale avec la méthodologie Smart*, Ministère de la Santé Publique et de la Population, UNICEF and WFP, Port-au-Prince, 2012.

77 Data provided by UNICEF Haiti, 2013.

78 United Nations Children's Fund, Global SAM Management Update, database accessed 1 October 2012.

79 Ayoya, Mohamed Ag, Kate Golden, Ismael Ngnie Teta, et al., 'Protecting and Improving Breastfeeding Practices during a Major Emergency: Lessons learnt from the baby tents in Haiti' (unpublished paper).

80 National Family Health Survey, 2005–2006, and UNICEF Global Databases.

81 Based on re-analysis of the National Family Health Survey, 2005–2006, and results of the Comprehensive Nutrition Survey in Maharashtra, 2012.

82 Comprehensive Nutrition Survey in Maharashtra, 2012.

83 Based on reanalysis of the National Family Health Survey, 2005–2006 and Comprehensive Nutrition Survey in Maharashtra, 2012.

84 World Bank, World Development Indicators, 2012.

85 United Nations Inter-agency Group for Child Mortality Estimation, 2012.

86 Demographic and Health Surveys, 2001 and 2011.

87 Demographic and Health Survey, 2011.

88 Ibid.

89 Ibid.

90 Ibid.

91 Demographic and Health Surveys, 1996, 2000, 2004–2006 and 2011.

92 Ibid.

93 Lechtig, Aaron, et al., 'Decreasing Stunting, Anemia, and Vitamin A Deficiency in Peru: Results of the Good Start in Life Program', *Food & Nutrition Bulletin*, vol. 30, no. 1, 2009, pp. 36–48.

94 Flores, Rosa, and Carlos Rojas, 'Impact of an Intervention on Food Security: REDESA program final evaluation', CARE Peru, Lima, 2007.

95 Demographic and Health Surveys, 1992 (reanalysed by UNICEF) and 2011.

96 United Nations Population Division 2010 data (reanalysed by UNICEF).

97 UNICEF Global Databases, 2012.

98 Demographic and Health Surveys, 2005 and 2010.

99 United Nations Children's Fund, 'UNICEF Humanitarian Action Update: Democratic Republic of the Congo', UNICEF, New York, 4 August 2012.

100 'Addressing a Silent and Unknown Crisis: Success in the treatment of severe acute malnutrition in the Democratic Republic of the Congo (DRC)' (internal document provided by UNICEF Democratic Republic of the Congo).

101 Ibid.

102 Ibid.

103 Ibid.

104 United Nations Children's Fund, Global SAM Management Update, database accessed 1 October 2012; United Nations Children's Fund, *UNICEF Humanitarian Action Update: Democratic Republic of the Congo*, UNICEF, New York, 4 August 2012, p. 7.

105 UNICEF Global Databases, 2012.

106 United Nations Inter-agency Group for Child Mortality Estimation, 2012.

107 Demographic and Health Survey, 2006–2007.

108 World Bank, 'Kyrgyz Republic Partnership: Program snapshot', World Bank, Washington, D.C., October 2012.

109 Research Institute of Obstetrics and Pediatrics (Kyrgyz Republic) and Macro International Inc., *Kyrgyz Republic Demographic and Health Survey, 1997*, Calverton, MD, 1998, pp. 128 and 132.

110 Lundeen, Elizabeth, et al., 'Daily Use of Sprinkles Micronutrient Powder for 2 Months Reduces Anemia among Children 6 to 36 Months of Age in the Kyrgyz Republic: A cluster-randomized trial', *Food & Nutrition Bulletin*, vol. 31, no. 3, September 2010, pp. 446–460.

111 Ministry of Health of Kyrgyz Republic, *Follow-up Survey of Nutritional Status in Children 6–24 Months of Age, Talas Oblast, Kyrgyz Republic 2010*, Ministry of Health of Kyrgyz Republic, Bishkek, 2011, p. 11.

112 United States Agency for International Development, 'Assessment of the Sustainability of the Tanzania National Vitamin A Supplementation Program: Results of a sustainability analysis', USAID, Washington, D.C., 2008, p. 5.

113 UNICEF Global Databases, 2012.

114 Masanja, Honorati, et al., 'Child Survival Gains in Tanzania: Analysis of data from demographic and health surveys', *Lancet*, vol. 371, no. 9620, 12 April 2008, pp. 1276–1283.

115 United Nations Inter-agency Group on Child Mortality Estimation, 2012.

116 UNICEF Global Databases, 2012.

117 Euromonitor International, 'Global Packaged Food: Market Opportunities for Baby Food to 2013', September 2008.

NUTRITION PROFILES

24 countries with the largest burden and highest prevalence of stunting

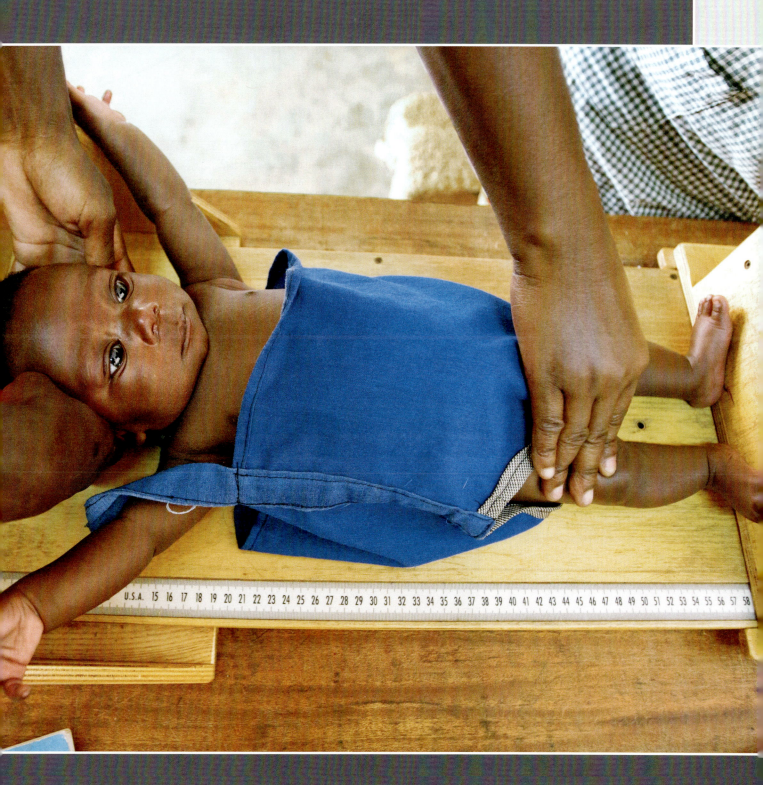

Bangladesh • Burundi • Central African Republic • China • Democratic Republic of the Congo • Ethiopia • Guatemala • Guinea • India • Indonesia • Liberia • Madagascar • Malawi • Mozambique • Nepal • Niger • Nigeria • Pakistan • Philippines • Rwanda • Sierra Leone • United Republic of Tanzania • Timor-Leste • Zambia

BANGLADESH

DEMOGRAPHICS AND BACKGROUND INFORMATION

Total population (000)	**150,494**	(2011)
Total under-five population (000)	**14,427**	(2011)
Total number of births (000)	**3,016**	(2011)
Under-five mortality rate (per 1,000 live births)	**46**	(2011)
Total number of under-five deaths (000)	**134**	(2011)
Infant mortality rate (per 1,000 live births)	**37**	(2011)
Neonatal mortality rate (per 1,000 live births)	**26**	(2011)
HIV prevalence rate (15–49 years old, %)	**<0.1**	(2011)
Population below international poverty line of US$1.25 per day (%)	**43**	(2011)
GNI per capita (US$)	**770**	(2011)
Primary school net attendance ratio (% female, % male)	**88, 85**	(2007)

Causes of under-five deaths, 2010
Globally, undernutrition contributes to more than one third of child deaths

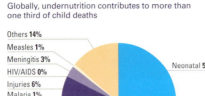
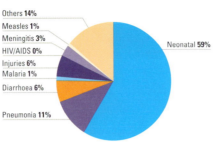

Others **14%**
Measles **1%**
Meningitis **3%**
HIV/AIDS **0%**
Injuries **6%**
Malaria **1%**
Diarrhoea **6%**
Pneumonia **11%**
Neonatal **59%**

Source: WHO/CHERG, 2012.

Under-five mortality rate
Deaths per 1,000 live births

139
46   46
MDG 4 target

Source: IGME, 2012.

NUTRITIONAL STATUS

Burden of malnutrition (2011)

Stunting country rank	**6**
Share of world stunting burden (%)	**4**

Stunted (under-fives, 000)	**5,958**
Wasted (under-fives, 000)	**2,251**
Severely wasted (under-fives, 000)	**577**

MDG 1 progress	**Insufficient progress**
Underweight (under-fives, 000)	**5,251**
Overweight (under-fives, 000)	**216**

Stunting trends
Percentage of children <5 years old stunted

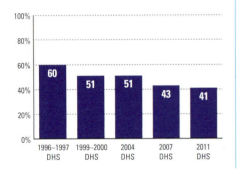

1996–1997 DHS	1999–2000 DHS	2004 DHS	2007 DHS	2011 DHS
60	51	51	43	41

Stunting disparities
Percentage of children <5 years old stunted, by selected background characteristics

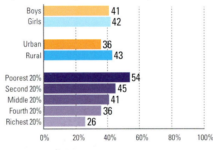

Boys 41
Girls 42
Urban 36
Rural 43
Poorest 20% 54
Second 20% 45
Middle 20% 41
Fourth 20% 36
Richest 20% 26

Source: DHS, 2011.

Underweight trends
Percentage of children <5 years old underweight

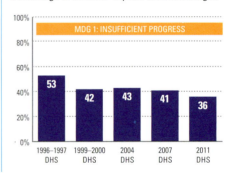

MDG 1: INSUFFICIENT PROGRESS

1996–1997 DHS	1999–2000 DHS	2004 DHS	2007 DHS	2011 DHS
53	42	43	41	36

INFANT AND YOUNG CHILD FEEDING

Exclusive breastfeeding trends
Percentage of infants <6 months old exclusively breastfed

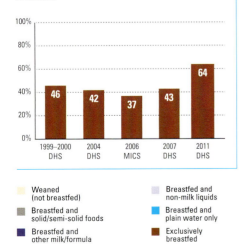

1999–2000 DHS	2004 DHS	2006 MICS	2007 DHS	2011 DHS
46	42	37	43	64

- Weaned (not breastfed)
- Breastfed and solid/semi-solid foods
- Breastfed and other milk/formula
- Breastfed and non-milk liquids
- Breastfed and plain water only
- Exclusively breastfed

Infant feeding practices, by age

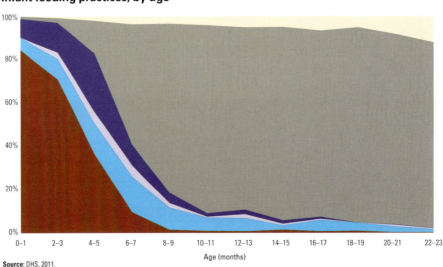

Age (months)

Source: DHS, 2011.

BANGLADESH

ESSENTIAL NUTRITION PRACTICES AND INTERVENTIONS DURING THE LIFE CYCLE

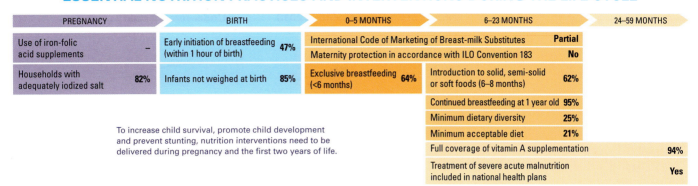

PREGNANCY	BIRTH	0–5 MONTHS	6–23 MONTHS	24–59 MONTHS

Use of iron-folic acid supplements	–	Early initiation of breastfeeding (within 1 hour of birth)	47%

International Code of Marketing of Breast-milk Substitutes	Partial
Maternity protection in accordance with ILO Convention 183	No

Households with adequately iodized salt	82%	Infants not weighed at birth	85%

Exclusive breastfeeding (<6 months)	64%

Introduction to solid, semi-solid or soft foods (6–8 months)	62%
Continued breastfeeding at 1 year old	95%
Minimum dietary diversity	25%
Minimum acceptable diet	21%

Full coverage of vitamin A supplementation	94%
Treatment of severe acute malnutrition included in national health plans	Yes

To increase child survival, promote child development and prevent stunting, nutrition interventions need to be delivered during pregnancy and the first two years of life.

MICRONUTRIENTS

Anaemia
Prevalence of anaemia among selected populations

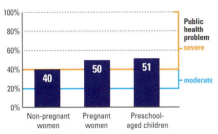

Source: DHS, 2011.

Iodized salt trends*
Percentage of households with adequately iodized salt
534,000 newborns are unprotected against iodine deficiency disorders (2011)

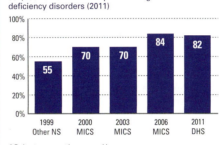

* Estimates may not be comparable.

Vitamin A supplementation
Percentage of children 6–59 months old receiving two doses of vitamin A during calendar year (full coverage)

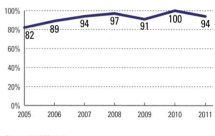

Source: UNICEF, 2012.

MATERNAL NUTRITION AND HEALTH

Maternal mortality ratio, adjusted (per 100,000 live births)	240	(2010)
Maternal mortality ratio, reported (per 100,000 live births)	220	(2010)
Total number of maternal deaths	7,200	(2010)
Lifetime risk of maternal death (1 in :)	170	(2010)
Women with low BMI (<18.5 kg/m², %)	24	(2011)
Anaemia, non-pregnant women (<120g/l, %)	40	(2011)
Antenatal care (at least one visit, %)	55	(2011)
Antenatal care (at least four visits, %)	26	(2011)
Skilled attendant at birth (%)	32	(2011)
Low birthweight (<2,500 grams, %)	22	(2006)
Women 20–24 years old who gave birth before age 18 (%)	40	(2007)

WATER AND SANITATION

Improved drinking water coverage
Percentage of population, by type of drinking water source, 1990–2010

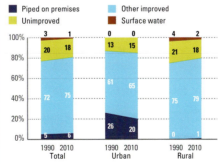

Source: WHO/UNICEF JMP, 2012.

Improved sanitation coverage
Percentage of population, by type of sanitation facility, 1990–2010

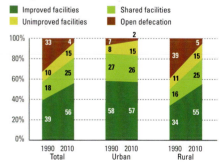

Source: WHO/UNICEF JMP, 2012.

DISPARITIES IN NUTRITION

Indicator	Gender			Residence			Wealth quintile						Equity chart	Source
	Male	Female	Ratio of male to female	Urban	Rural	Ratio of urban to rural	Poorest	Second	Middle	Fourth	Richest	Ratio of richest to poorest		
Stunting prevalence (%)	41	42	1.0	36	43	0.8	54	45	41	36	26	0.5	▪▪▪▪▪	DHS, 2011
Underweight prevalence (%)	34	39	0.9	28	39	0.7	50	42	36	28	21	0.4	▪▪▪▪▪	DHS, 2011
Wasting prevalence (%)	16	15	1.1	14	16	0.9	18	16	18	14	12	0.7	▬▬▬▬▬	DHS, 2011
Women with low BMI (<18.5 kg/m², %)	–	24	–	14	28	0.5	40	30	26	20	8	0.2	▪▪▪▪▬	DHS, 2011
Women with high BMI (≥25 kg/m², %)	–	17	–	29	12	2.4	5	7	11	20	37	7.3	▬▬▬▬▪	DHS, 2011

BURUNDI

DEMOGRAPHICS AND BACKGROUND INFORMATION

Total population (000)	**8,575**	(2011)
Total under-five population (000)	**1,218**	(2011)
Total number of births (000)	**288**	(2011)
Under-five mortality rate (per 1,000 live births)	**139**	(2011)
Total number of under-five deaths (000)	**39**	(2011)
Infant mortality rate (per 1,000 live births)	**86**	(2011)
Neonatal mortality rate (per 1,000 live births)	**43**	(2011)
HIV prevalence rate (15–49 years old, %)	**1.3**	(2011)
Population below international poverty line of US$1.25 per day (%)	**81**	(2006)
GNI per capita (US$)	**250**	(2011)
Primary school net attendance ratio (% female, % male)	**74, 73**	(2010)

Causes of under-five deaths, 2010
Globally, undernutrition contributes to more than one third of child deaths

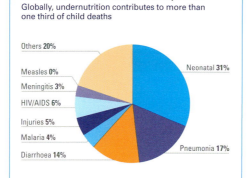

Others **20%**
Neonatal **31%**
Measles **0%**
Meningitis **3%**
HIV/AIDS **6%**
Injuries **5%**
Malaria **4%**
Pneumonia **17%**
Diarrhoea **14%**

Source: WHO/CHERG, 2012.

Under-five mortality rate
Deaths per 1,000 live births

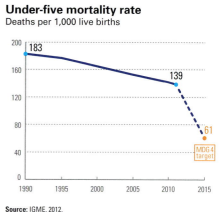

Source: IGME, 2012.

NUTRITIONAL STATUS

Burden of malnutrition (2011)

Stunting country rank	**33**
Share of world stunting burden (%)	**<1%**

Stunted (under-fives, 000)	**703**
Wasted (under-fives, 000)	**71**
Severely wasted (under-fives, 000)	**17**

MDG 1 progress	**No progress**
Underweight (under-fives, 000)	**351**
Overweight (under-fives, 000)	**33**

Stunting trends
Percentage of children <5 years old stunted

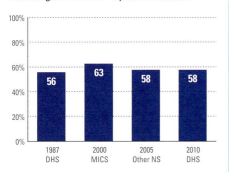

Stunting disparities
Percentage of children <5 years old stunted, by selected background characteristics

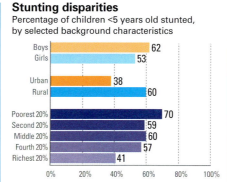

Boys 62
Girls 53
Urban 38
Rural 60
Poorest 20% 70
Second 20% 59
Middle 20% 60
Fourth 20% 57
Richest 20% 41

Source: DHS, 2010.

Underweight trends
Percentage of children <5 years old underweight

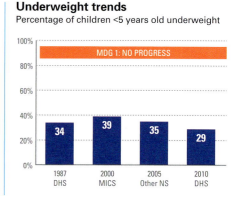

INFANT AND YOUNG CHILD FEEDING

Exclusive breastfeeding trends
Percentage of infants <6 months old exclusively breastfed

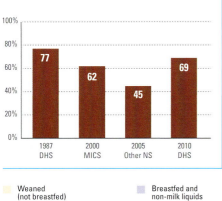

 Weaned (not breastfed)
Breastfed and solid/semi-solid foods
Breastfed and other milk/formula
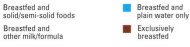 Breastfed and non-milk liquids
Breastfed and plain water only
Exclusively breastfed

Infant feeding practices, by age

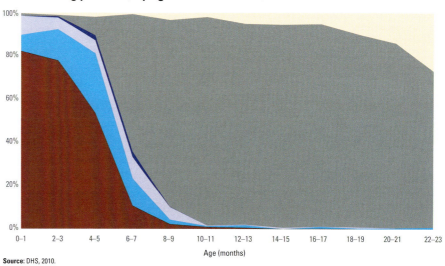

Age (months)

Source: DHS, 2010.

BURUNDI

ESSENTIAL NUTRITION PRACTICES AND INTERVENTIONS DURING THE LIFE CYCLE

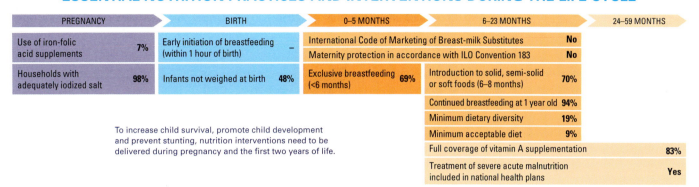

PREGNANCY	BIRTH	0–5 MONTHS	6–23 MONTHS	24–59 MONTHS

Use of iron-folic acid supplements	**7%**	
Households with adequately iodized salt	**98%**	

Early initiation of breastfeeding (within 1 hour of birth)	**–**
Infants not weighed at birth	**48%**

International Code of Marketing of Breast-milk Substitutes	**No**
Maternity protection in accordance with ILO Convention 183	**No**
Exclusive breastfeeding (<6 months)	**69%**

Introduction to solid, semi-solid or soft foods (6–8 months)	**70%**
Continued breastfeeding at 1 year old	**94%**
Minimum dietary diversity	**19%**
Minimum acceptable diet	**9%**
Full coverage of vitamin A supplementation	**83%**
Treatment of severe acute malnutrition included in national health plans	**Yes**

To increase child survival, promote child development and prevent stunting, nutrition interventions need to be delivered during pregnancy and the first two years of life.

MICRONUTRIENTS

Anaemia
Prevalence of anaemia among selected populations

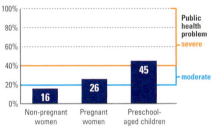

Non-pregnant women: 16
Pregnant women: 26
Preschool-aged children: 45

Public health problem – severe / moderate

Source: DHS, 2010.

Iodized salt trends*
Percentage of households with adequately iodized salt

6,000 newborns are unprotected against iodine deficiency disorders (2011)

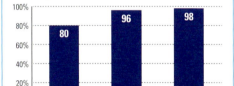

1993 UNICEF: 80
2000 MICS: 96
2005 Other NS: 98

* Estimates may not be comparable.

Vitamin A supplementation
Percentage of children 6–59 months old receiving two doses of vitamin A during calendar year (full coverage)

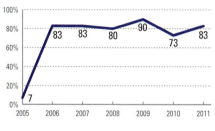

2005: 7
2006: 83
2007: 83
2008: 80
2009: 90
2010: 73
2011: 83

Source: UNICEF, 2012.

MATERNAL NUTRITION AND HEALTH

Maternal mortality ratio, adjusted (per 100,000 live births)	800	(2010)
Maternal mortality ratio, reported (per 100,000 live births)	500	(2010)
Total number of maternal deaths	2,200	(2010)
Lifetime risk of maternal death (1 in :)	31	(2010)
Women with low BMI (<18.5 kg/m², %)	16	(2010)
Anaemia, non-pregnant women (<120g/l, %)	16	(2010)
Antenatal care (at least one visit, %)	99	(2010)
Antenatal care (at least four visits, %)	33	(2010)
Skilled attendant at birth (%)	60	(2010)
Low birthweight (<2,500 grams, %)	11	(2005)
Women 20–24 years old who gave birth before age 18 (%)	11	(2010)

WATER AND SANITATION

Improved drinking water coverage
Percentage of population, by type of drinking water source, 1990–2010

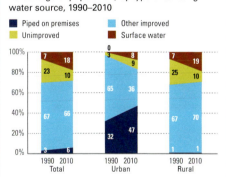

Legend: Piped on premises / Other improved / Unimproved / Surface water

Source: WHO/UNICEF JMP, 2012.

Improved sanitation coverage
Percentage of population, by type of sanitation facility, 1990–2010

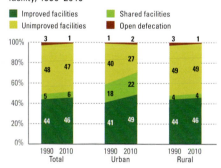

Legend: Improved facilities / Shared facilities / Unimproved facilities / Open defecation

Source: WHO/UNICEF JMP, 2012.

DISPARITIES IN NUTRITION

Indicator	Gender			Residence			Wealth quintile							Source
	Male	Female	Ratio of male to female	Urban	Rural	Ratio of urban to rural	Poorest	Second	Middle	Fourth	Richest	Ratio of richest to poorest	Equity chart	
Stunting prevalence (%)	62	53	1.2	38	60	0.6	70	59	60	57	41	0.6	▪▪▪▪▫	DHS, 2010
Underweight prevalence (%)	32	26	1.2	18	30	0.6	41	30	30	25	17	0.4	▪▪▫▫▫	DHS, 2010
Wasting prevalence (%)	6	6	1.1	5	6	0.8	7	6	5	5	5	0.8	▫▫▫▫▫	DHS, 2010
Women with low BMI (<18.5 kg/m², %)	–	16	–	10	17	0.6	22	15	17	15	12	0.5	▫▫▫▫▫	DHS, 2010
Women with high BMI (≥25 kg/m², %)	–	8	–	27	5	5.3	4	3	6	6	19	5.4	▫▫▫▫▪	DHS, 2010

CENTRAL AFRICAN REPUBLIC

DEMOGRAPHICS AND BACKGROUND INFORMATION

Total population (000)	**4,487**	(2011)
Total under-five population (000)	**659**	(2011)
Total number of births (000)	**156**	(2011)
Under-five mortality rate (per 1,000 live births)	**164**	(2011)
Total number of under-five deaths (000)	**25**	(2011)
Infant mortality rate (per 1,000 live births)	**108**	(2011)
Neonatal mortality rate (per 1,000 live births)	**46**	(2011)
HIV prevalence rate (15–49 years old, %)	**4.6**	(2011)
Population below international poverty line of US$1.25 per day (%)	**63**	(2008)
GNI per capita (US$)	**470**	(2011)
Primary school net attendance ratio (% female, % male)	**47, 56**	(2006)

Causes of under-five deaths, 2010
Globally, undernutrition contributes to more than one third of child deaths

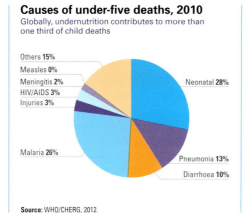

Others 15%
Measles 0%
Meningitis 2%
HIV/AIDS 3%
Injuries 3%
Neonatal 28%
Malaria 26%
Pneumonia 13%
Diarrhoea 10%

Source: WHO/CHERG, 2012.

Under-five mortality rate
Deaths per 1,000 live births

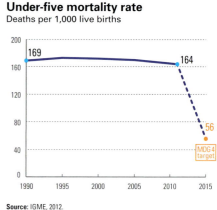

Source: IGME, 2012.

NUTRITIONAL STATUS

Burden of malnutrition (2011)

Stunting country rank	**50**
Share of world stunting burden (%)	**<1%**

Stunted (under-fives, 000)	**270**
Wasted (under-fives, 000)	**46**
Severely wasted (under-fives, 000)	**13**

MDG 1 progress	**No progress**
Underweight (under-fives, 000)	**158**
Overweight (under-fives, 000)	**12**

Stunting trends
Percentage of children <5 years old stunted

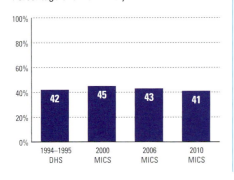

1994–1995 DHS	2000 MICS	2006 MICS	2010 MICS
42	45	43	41

Stunting disparities
Percentage of children <5 years old stunted, by selected background characteristics

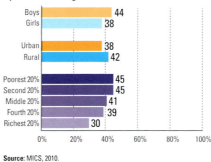

Boys	44
Girls	38
Urban	38
Rural	42
Poorest 20%	45
Second 20%	45
Middle 20%	41
Fourth 20%	39
Richest 20%	30

Source: MICS, 2010.

Underweight trends
Percentage of children <5 years old underweight

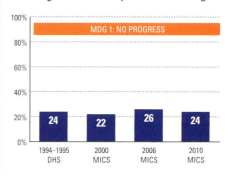

MDG 1: NO PROGRESS

1994–1995 DHS	2000 MICS	2006 MICS	2010 MICS
24	22	26	24

INFANT AND YOUNG CHILD FEEDING

Exclusive breastfeeding trends
Percentage of infants <6 months old exclusively breastfed

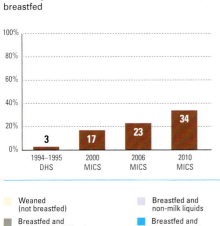

1994–1995 DHS	2000 MICS	2006 MICS	2010 MICS
3	17	23	34

Infant feeding practices, by age

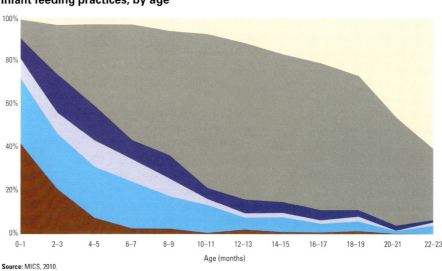

- Weaned (not breastfed)
- Breastfed and solid/semi-solid foods
- Breastfed and other milk/formula
- Breastfed and non-milk liquids
- Breastfed and plain water only
- Exclusively breastfed

Age (months)

Source: MICS, 2010.

CENTRAL AFRICAN REPUBLIC

ESSENTIAL NUTRITION PRACTICES AND INTERVENTIONS DURING THE LIFE CYCLE

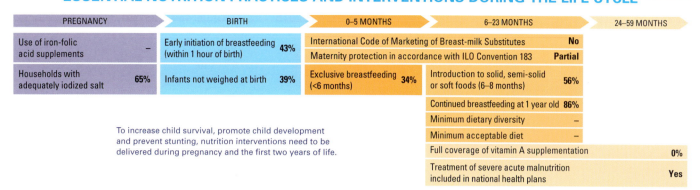

PREGNANCY	BIRTH	0–5 MONTHS	6–23 MONTHS	24–59 MONTHS

Use of iron-folic acid supplements	–	Early initiation of breastfeeding (within 1 hour of birth) **43%**
Households with adequately iodized salt	**65%**	Infants not weighed at birth **39%**

International Code of Marketing of Breast-milk Substitutes	**No**
Maternity protection in accordance with ILO Convention 183	**Partial**

Exclusive breastfeeding (<6 months) **34%**

Introduction to solid, semi-solid or soft foods (6–8 months)	**56%**
Continued breastfeeding at 1 year old	**86%**
Minimum dietary diversity	–
Minimum acceptable diet	–
Full coverage of vitamin A supplementation	**0%**
Treatment of severe acute malnutrition included in national health plans	**Yes**

To increase child survival, promote child development and prevent stunting, nutrition interventions need to be delivered during pregnancy and the first two years of life.

MICRONUTRIENTS

Anaemia
Prevalence of anaemia among selected populations

NO DATA

Iodized salt trends*
Percentage of households with adequately iodized salt

55,000 newborns are unprotected against iodine deficiency disorders (2011)

Bar chart:
- 1998 Other NS: 87
- 2000 MICS: 86
- 2006 MICS: 62
- 2010 MICS: 65

*Estimates may not be comparable.

Vitamin A supplementation
Percentage of children 6–59 months old receiving two doses of vitamin A during calendar year (full coverage)

Line chart:
- 2005: 76
- 2006: 8
- 2007: 78
- 2008: 68
- 2009: 87
- 2010: 0
- 2011: 0

Source: UNICEF, 2012.

MATERNAL NUTRITION AND HEALTH

Maternal mortality ratio, adjusted (per 100,000 live births)	890	(2010)
Maternal mortality ratio, reported (per 100,000 live births)	540	(2006)
Total number of maternal deaths	1,400	(2010)
Lifetime risk of maternal death (1 in :)	26	(2010)
Women with low BMI (<18.5 kg/m², %)	–	–
Anaemia, non-pregnant women (<120g/l, %)	–	–
Antenatal care (at least one visit, %)	68	(2010)
Antenatal care (at least four visits, %)	38	(2010)
Skilled attendant at birth (%)	54	(2010)
Low birthweight (<2,500 grams, %)	14	(2010)
Women 20–24 years old who gave birth before age 18 (%)	45	(2010)

WATER AND SANITATION

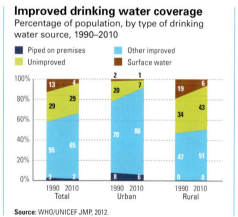

Improved drinking water coverage
Percentage of population, by type of drinking water source, 1990–2010

Legend: Piped on premises / Other improved / Unimproved / Surface water

Total 1990: 3, 55, 29, 13
Total 2010: 2, 65, 29, 4
Urban 1990: 8, 70, 20, 2
Urban 2010: 6, 86, 7, 1
Rural 1990: 0, 47, 34, 19
Rural 2010: 0, 51, 43, 6

Source: WHO/UNICEF JMP, 2012.

Improved sanitation coverage
Percentage of population, by type of sanitation facility, 1990–2010

Legend: Improved facilities / Shared facilities / Unimproved facilities / Open defecation

Total 1990: 11, 6, 48, 35
Total 2010: 34, 18, 28, 20
Urban 1990: 21, 12, 57, 10
Urban 2010: 43, 24, 30, 3
Rural 1990: 5, 44, 49
Rural 2010: 2, 28, 14, 27, 31

Source: WHO/UNICEF JMP, 2012.

DISPARITIES IN NUTRITION

Indicator	Gender			Residence			Wealth quintile							Source
	Male	Female	Ratio of male to female	Urban	Rural	Ratio of urban to rural	Poorest	Second	Middle	Fourth	Richest	Ratio of richest to poorest	Equity chart	
Stunting prevalence (%)	44	38	1.2	38	42	0.9	45	45	41	39	30	0.7	▪▪▪▪▪	MICS, 2010
Underweight prevalence (%)	26	21	1.2	23	24	1.0	26	25	22	24	19	0.7	▪▪▪▪▪	MICS, 2010
Wasting prevalence (%)	9	6	1.5	8	7	1.1	8	7	6	8	9	1.1	▬▬▬▬▬	MICS, 2010
Women with low BMI (<18.5 kg/m², %)	–	–	–	–	–	–	–	–	–	–	–	–		–
Women with high BMI (≥25 kg/m², %)	–	–	–	–	–	–	–	–	–	–	–	–		–

CHINA

DEMOGRAPHICS AND BACKGROUND INFORMATION

Total population (000)	**1,347,565** (2011)
Total under-five population (000)	**82,231** (2011)
Total number of births (000)	**16,364** (2011)
Under-five mortality rate (per 1,000 live births)	**15** (2011)
Total number of under-five deaths (000)	**249** (2011)
Infant mortality rate (per 1,000 live births)	**13** (2011)
Neonatal mortality rate (per 1,000 live births)	**9** (2011)
HIV prevalence rate (15–49 years old, %)	– –
Population below international poverty line of US$1.25 per day (%)	**13** (2008)
GNI per capita (US$)	**4,930** (2011)
Primary school net attendance ratio (% female, % male)	– –

Causes of under-five deaths, 2010
Globally, undernutrition contributes to more than one third of child deaths

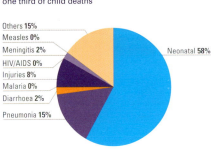

Others 15%
Measles 0%
Meningitis 2%
HIV/AIDS 0%
Injuries 8%
Malaria 0%
Diarrhoea 2%
Pneumonia 15%
Neonatal **58%**

Source: WHO/CHERG, 2012.

Under-five mortality rate
Deaths per 1,000 live births

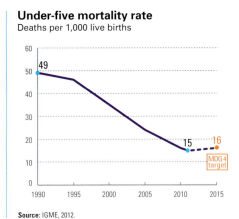

Source: IGME, 2012.

NUTRITIONAL STATUS

Burden of malnutrition (2011)

Stunting country rank	**4**
Share of world stunting burden (%)	**5**

Stunted (under-fives, 000)	**8,059**	
Wasted (under-fives, 000)	**1,891**	
Severely wasted (under-fives, 000)	–	

MDG 1 progress	**On track**	
Underweight (under-fives, 000)	**2,960**	
Overweight (under-fives, 000)	**5,427**	

Stunting trends
Percentage of children <5 years old stunted

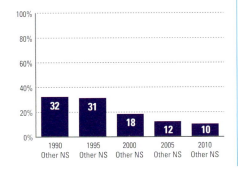

Stunting disparities
Percentage of children <5 years old stunted, by selected background characteristics

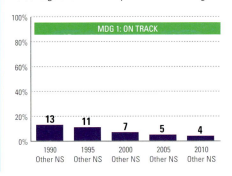

Boys
Girls
Urban 3
Rural 12
Poorest 20%
Second 20%
Middle 20%
Fourth 20%
Richest 20%

Source: Other NS, 2010.

Underweight trends
Percentage of children <5 years old underweight

MDG 1: ON TRACK

13 11 7 5 4

1990 Other NS 1995 Other NS 2000 Other NS 2005 Other NS 2010 Other NS

INFANT AND YOUNG CHILD FEEDING

Exclusive breastfeeding trends
Percentage of infants <6 months old exclusively breastfed

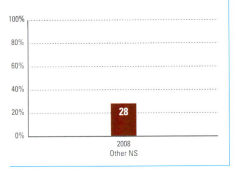

28

2008 Other NS

Infant feeding practices, by age

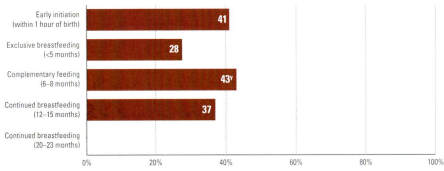

Early initiation (within 1 hour of birth) — 41
Exclusive breastfeeding (<5 months) — 28
Complementary feeding (6–8 months) — 43ʸ
Continued breastfeeding (12–15 months) — 37
Continued breastfeeding (20–23 months)

Source: Other NS, 2008.

ESSENTIAL NUTRITION PRACTICES AND INTERVENTIONS DURING THE LIFE CYCLE

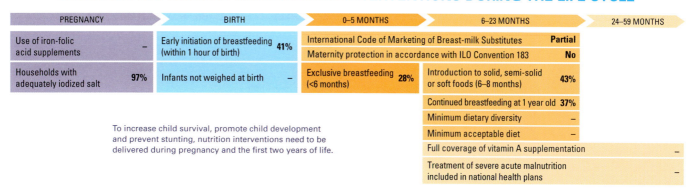

PREGNANCY	BIRTH	0–5 MONTHS	6–23 MONTHS	24–59 MONTHS

Use of iron-folic acid supplements	–	Early initiation of breastfeeding (within 1 hour of birth)	**41%**
Households with adequately iodized salt	**97%**	Infants not weighed at birth	–

International Code of Marketing of Breast-milk Substitutes	**Partial**
Maternity protection in accordance with ILO Convention 183	**No**

Exclusive breastfeeding (<6 months)	**28%**

Introduction to solid, semi-solid or soft foods (6–8 months)	**43%**
Continued breastfeeding at 1 year old	**37%**
Minimum dietary diversity	–
Minimum acceptable diet	–
Full coverage of vitamin A supplementation	–
Treatment of severe acute malnutrition included in national health plans	–

To increase child survival, promote child development and prevent stunting, nutrition interventions need to be delivered during pregnancy and the first two years of life.

MICRONUTRIENTS

Anaemia
Prevalence of anaemia among selected populations

NO DATA

Iodized salt trends*
Percentage of households with adequately iodized salt

524,000 newborns are unprotected against iodine deficiency disorders (2011)

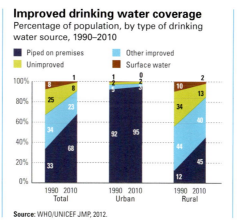

1995 Other NS	60
2002 Other NS	93
2008 Other NS	95
2011 Other NS	97

* Estimates may not be comparable.

Vitamin A supplementation
Percentage of children 6–59 months old receiving two doses of vitamin A during calendar year (full coverage)

NO DATA

MATERNAL NUTRITION AND HEALTH

Maternal mortality ratio, adjusted (per 100,000 live births)	**37**	(2010)
Maternal mortality ratio, reported (per 100,000 live births)	**30**	(2010)
Total number of maternal deaths	**6,000**	(2010)
Lifetime risk of maternal death (1 in :)	**1,700**	(2010)
Women with low BMI (<18.5 kg/m², %)	–	–
Anaemia, non-pregnant women (<120g/l, %)	–	–
Antenatal care (at least one visit, %)	**94**	(2010)
Antenatal care (at least four visits, %)	–	–
Skilled attendant at birth (%)	**100**	(2010)
Low birthweight (<2,500 grams, %)	**3**	(2008)
Women 20–24 years old who gave birth before age 18 (%)	–	–

WATER AND SANITATION

Improved drinking water coverage
Percentage of population, by type of drinking water source, 1990–2010

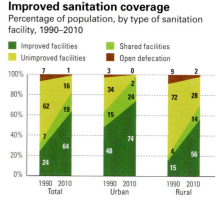

- Piped on premises
- Other improved
- Unimproved
- Surface water

Source: WHO/UNICEF JMP, 2012.

Improved sanitation coverage
Percentage of population, by type of sanitation facility, 1990–2010

- Improved facilities
- Shared facilities
- Unimproved facilities
- Open defecation

Source: WHO/UNICEF JMP, 2012.

DISPARITIES IN NUTRITION

Indicator	Gender			Residence			Wealth quintile							Source
	Male	Female	Ratio of male to female	Urban	Rural	Ratio of urban to rural	Poorest	Second	Middle	Fourth	Richest	Ratio of richest to poorest	Equity chart	
Stunting prevalence (%)	–	–	–	3	12	0.3	–	–	–	–	–	–		Other NS, 2010
Underweight prevalence (%)	–	–	–	1	4	0.3	–	–	–	–	–	–		Other NS, 2010
Wasting prevalence (%)	–	–	–	–	–	–	–	–	–	–	–	–		–
Women with low BMI (<18.5 kg/m², %)	–	–	–	–	–	–	–	–	–	–	–	–		–
Women with high BMI (≥25 kg/m², %)	–	–	–	–	–	–	–	–	–	–	–	–		–

DEMOCRATIC REPUBLIC OF THE CONGO

DEMOGRAPHICS AND BACKGROUND INFORMATION

Total population (000)	**67,758**	(2011)
Total under-five population (000)	**12,046**	(2011)
Total number of births (000)	**2,912**	(2011)
Under-five mortality rate (per 1,000 live births)	**168**	(2011)
Total number of under-five deaths (000)	**465**	(2011)
Infant mortality rate (per 1,000 live births)	**111**	(2011)
Neonatal mortality rate (per 1,000 live births)	**47**	(2011)
HIV prevalence rate (15–49 years old, %)	–	–
Population below international poverty line of US$1.25 per day (%)	**88**	(2006)
GNI per capita (US$)	**190**	(2011)
Primary school net attendance ratio (% female, % male)	**72, 78**	(2010)

Causes of under-five deaths, 2010
Globally, undernutrition contributes to more than one third of child deaths

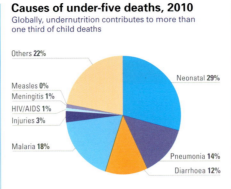

Others 22%
Neonatal 29%
Measles 0%
Meningitis 1%
HIV/AIDS 1%
Injuries 3%
Malaria 18%
Pneumonia 14%
Diarrhoea 12%

Source: WHO/CHERG, 2012.

Under-five mortality rate
Deaths per 1,000 live births

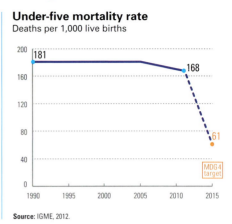

181
168
61
MDG 4 target

Source: IGME, 2012.

NUTRITIONAL STATUS

Burden of malnutrition (2011)

Stunting country rank	**8**
Share of world stunting burden (%)	**3**

Stunted (under-fives, 000)	**5,228**	MDG 1 progress	**Insufficient progress**
Wasted (under-fives, 000)	**1,024**	Underweight (under-fives, 000)	**2,915**
Severely wasted (under-fives, 000)	**337**	Overweight (under-fives, 000)	–

Stunting trends
Percentage of children <5 years old stunted

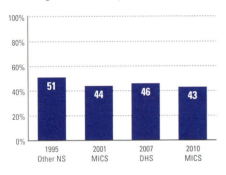

1995 Other NS	2001 MICS	2007 DHS	2010 MICS
51	44	46	43

Stunting disparities
Percentage of children <5 years old stunted, by selected background characteristics

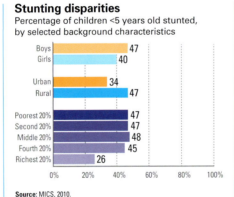

Boys	47
Girls	40
Urban	34
Rural	47
Poorest 20%	47
Second 20%	47
Middle 20%	48
Fourth 20%	45
Richest 20%	26

Source: MICS, 2010.

Underweight trends
Percentage of children <5 years old underweight

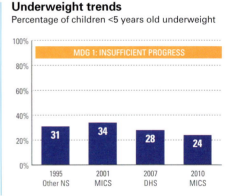

MDG 1: INSUFFICIENT PROGRESS

1995 Other NS	2001 MICS	2007 DHS	2010 MICS
31	34	28	24

INFANT AND YOUNG CHILD FEEDING

Exclusive breastfeeding trends
Percentage of infants <6 months old exclusively breastfed

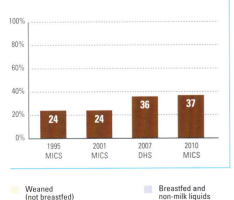

1995 MICS	2001 MICS	2007 DHS	2010 MICS
24	24	36	37

Infant feeding practices, by age

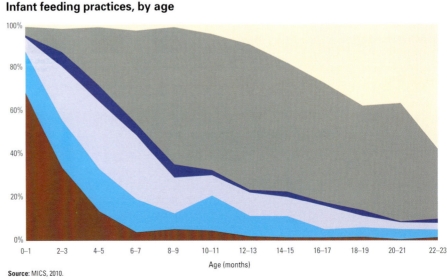

Age (months)

Weaned (not breastfed)
Breastfed and solid/semi-solid foods
Breastfed and other milk/formula
Breastfed and non-milk liquids
Breastfed and plain water only
Exclusively breastfed

Source: MICS, 2010.

DEMOCRATIC REPUBLIC OF THE CONGO

ESSENTIAL NUTRITION PRACTICES AND INTERVENTIONS DURING THE LIFE CYCLE

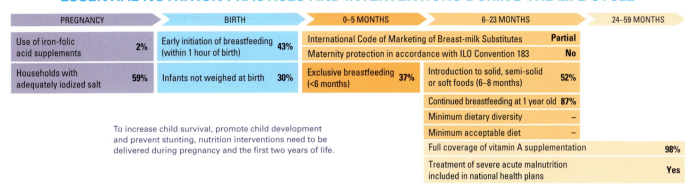

PREGNANCY	BIRTH	0–5 MONTHS	6–23 MONTHS	24–59 MONTHS

Use of iron-folic acid supplements	**2%**	
Households with adequately iodized salt	**59%**	

Early initiation of breastfeeding (within 1 hour of birth)	**43%**
Infants not weighed at birth	**30%**

International Code of Marketing of Breast-milk Substitutes	**Partial**
Maternity protection in accordance with ILO Convention 183	**No**
Exclusive breastfeeding (<6 months)	**37%**
Introduction to solid, semi-solid or soft foods (6–8 months)	**52%**
Continued breastfeeding at 1 year old	**87%**
Minimum dietary diversity	**–**
Minimum acceptable diet	**–**
Full coverage of vitamin A supplementation	**98%**
Treatment of severe acute malnutrition included in national health plans	**Yes**

To increase child survival, promote child development and prevent stunting, nutrition interventions need to be delivered during pregnancy and the first two years of life.

MICRONUTRIENTS

Anaemia
Prevalence of anaemia among selected populations

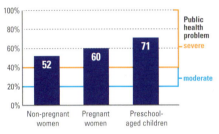

Source: DHS, 2007.

Iodized salt trends*
Percentage of households with adequately iodized salt

1,206,000 newborns are unprotected against iodine deficiency disorders (2011)

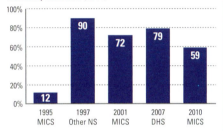

* Estimates may not be comparable.

Vitamin A supplementation
Percentage of children 6–59 months old receiving two doses of vitamin A during calendar year (full coverage)

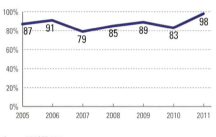

Source: UNICEF, 2012.

MATERNAL NUTRITION AND HEALTH

Maternal mortality ratio, adjusted (per 100,000 live births)	**540**	(2010)
Maternal mortality ratio, reported (per 100,000 live births)	**550**	(2007)
Total number of maternal deaths	**15,000**	(2010)
Lifetime risk of maternal death (1 in :)	**30**	(2010)
Women with low BMI (<18.5 kg/m², %)	**19**	(2007)
Anaemia, non-pregnant women (<120g/l, %)	**52**	(2007)
Antenatal care (at least one visit, %)	**89**	(2010)
Antenatal care (at least four visits, %)	**45**	(2010)
Skilled attendant at birth (%)	**80**	(2010)
Low birthweight (<2,500 grams, %)	**10**	(2010)
Women 20–24 years old who gave birth before age 18 (%)	**25**	(2010)

WATER AND SANITATION

Improved drinking water coverage
Percentage of population, by type of drinking water source, 1990–2010

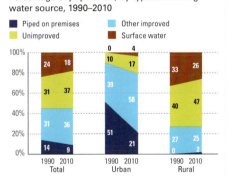

Source: WHO/UNICEF JMP, 2012.

Improved sanitation coverage
Percentage of population, by type of sanitation facility, 1990–2010

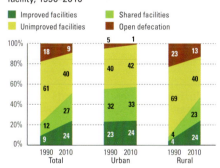

Source: WHO/UNICEF JMP, 2012.

DISPARITIES IN NUTRITION

Indicator	Gender			Residence			Wealth quintile						Equity chart	Source
	Male	Female	Ratio of male to female	Urban	Rural	Ratio of urban to rural	Poorest	Second	Middle	Fourth	Richest	Ratio of richest to poorest		
Stunting prevalence (%)	47	40	1.2	34	47	0.7	47	47	48	45	26	0.6	▪▪▪▪▫	MICS, 2010
Underweight prevalence (%)	27	21	1.3	17	27	0.6	29	28	27	21	12	0.4	▪▪▪▪▫	MICS, 2010
Wasting prevalence (%)	10	8	1.3	7	9	0.8	10	9	10	6	7	0.7	▫▫▫▫▫	MICS, 2010
Women with low BMI (<18.5 kg/m², %)	–	19	–	16	21	0.8	23	20	21	15	15	0.7	▪▪▪▪▫	DHS, 2007
Women with high BMI (≥25 kg/m², %)	–	11	–	18	6	2.9	6	6	7	13	23	3.8	▫▫▫▫▪	DHS, 2007

ETHIOPIA

Total population (000)	**84,734**	(2011)
Total under-five population (000)	**11,918**	(2011)
Total number of births (000)	**2,613**	(2011)
Under-five mortality rate (per 1,000 live births)	**77**	(2011)
Total number of under-five deaths (000)	**194**	(2011)
Infant mortality rate (per 1,000 live births)	**52**	(2011)
Neonatal mortality rate (per 1,000 live births)	**31**	(2011)
HIV prevalence rate (15–49 years old, %)	**1.4**	(2011)
Population below international poverty line of US$1.25 per day (%)	**39**	(2005)
GNI per capita (US$)	**400**	(2011)
Primary school net attendance ratio (% female, % male)	**65, 64**	(2011)

Causes of under-five deaths, 2010
Globally, undernutrition contributes to more than one third of child deaths

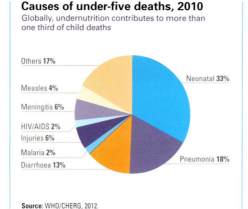

Others 17%
Measles 4%
Meningitis 6%
HIV/AIDS 2%
Injuries 6%
Malaria 2%
Diarrhoea 13%
Neonatal 33%
Pneumonia 18%

Source: WHO/CHERG, 2012.

Under-five mortality rate
Deaths per 1,000 live births

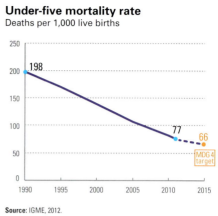

Source: IGME, 2012.

NUTRITIONAL STATUS

Burden of malnutrition (2011)

Stunting country rank	**7**
Share of world stunting burden (%)	**3**

Stunted (under-fives, 000)	**5,291**
Wasted (under-fives, 000)	**1,156**
Severely wasted (under-fives, 000)	**334**

MDG 1 progress	**Insufficient progress**
Underweight (under-fives, 000)	**3,420**
Overweight (under-fives, 000)	**203**

Stunting trends
Percentage of children <5 years old stunted

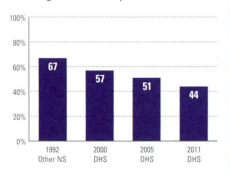

1992 Other NS	2000 DHS	2005 DHS	2011 DHS
67	57	51	44

Stunting disparities
Percentage of children <5 years old stunted, by selected background characteristics

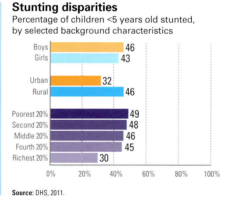

Boys 46
Girls 43
Urban 32
Rural 46
Poorest 20% 49
Second 20% 48
Middle 20% 46
Fourth 20% 45
Richest 20% 30

Source: DHS, 2011.

Underweight trends
Percentage of children <5 years old underweight

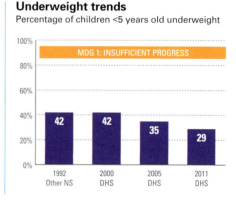

MDG 1: INSUFFICIENT PROGRESS

1992 Other NS	2000 DHS	2005 DHS	2011 DHS
42	42	35	29

INFANT AND YOUNG CHILD FEEDING

Exclusive breastfeeding trends
Percentage of infants <6 months old exclusively breastfed

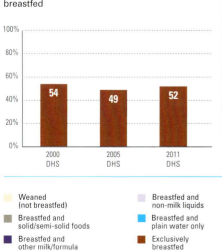

2000 DHS	2005 DHS	2011 DHS
54	49	52

Weaned (not breastfed)

Breastfed and solid/semi-solid foods

Breastfed and other milk/formula

Breastfed and non-milk liquids

Breastfed and plain water only

Exclusively breastfed

Infant feeding practices, by age

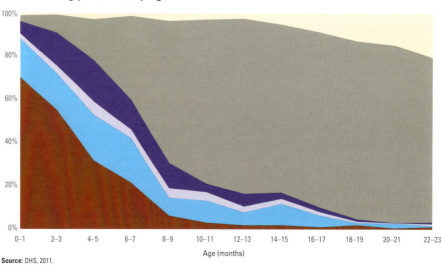

Age (months)

Source: DHS, 2011.

ESSENTIAL NUTRITION PRACTICES AND INTERVENTIONS DURING THE LIFE CYCLE

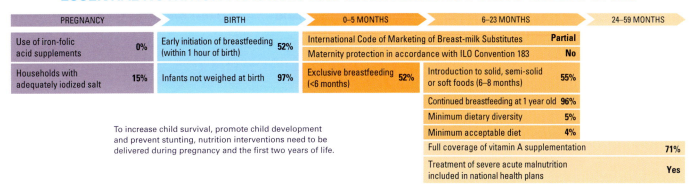

| PREGNANCY | BIRTH | 0–5 MONTHS | 6–23 MONTHS | 24–59 MONTHS |

Use of iron-folic acid supplements	0%
Households with adequately iodized salt	15%

Early initiation of breastfeeding (within 1 hour of birth)	52%
Infants not weighed at birth	97%

International Code of Marketing of Breast-milk Substitutes	Partial
Maternity protection in accordance with ILO Convention 183	No
Exclusive breastfeeding (<6 months)	52%

Introduction to solid, semi-solid or soft foods (6–8 months)	55%
Continued breastfeeding at 1 year old	96%
Minimum dietary diversity	5%
Minimum acceptable diet	4%
Full coverage of vitamin A supplementation	71%
Treatment of severe acute malnutrition included in national health plans	Yes

To increase child survival, promote child development and prevent stunting, nutrition interventions need to be delivered during pregnancy and the first two years of life.

MICRONUTRIENTS

Anaemia
Prevalence of anaemia among selected populations

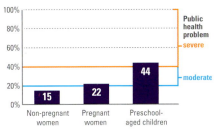

Non-pregnant women: 15
Pregnant women: 22
Preschool-aged children: 44

Public health problem — severe / moderate

Source: DHS, 2011.

Iodized salt trends*
Percentage of households with adequately iodized salt

2,211,000 newborns are unprotected against iodine deficiency disorders (2011)

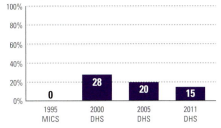

1995 MICS: 0
2000 DHS: 28
2005 DHS: 20
2011 DHS: 15

* Estimates may not be comparable.

Vitamin A supplementation
Percentage of children 6–59 months old receiving two doses of vitamin A during calendar year (full coverage)

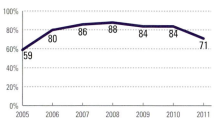

2005: 59
2006: 80
2007: 86
2008: 88
2009: 84
2010: 84
2011: 71

Source: UNICEF, 2012.

MATERNAL NUTRITION AND HEALTH

Maternal mortality ratio, adjusted (per 100,000 live births)	350	(2010)
Maternal mortality ratio, reported (per 100,000 live births)	680	(2011)
Total number of maternal deaths	9,000	(2010)
Lifetime risk of maternal death (1 in :)	67	(2010)
Women with low BMI (<18.5 kg/m², %)	27	(2011)
Anaemia, non-pregnant women (<120g/l, %)	15	(2011)
Antenatal care (at least one visit, %)	43	(2011)
Antenatal care (at least four visits, %)	19	(2011)
Skilled attendant at birth (%)	10	(2011)
Low birthweight (<2,500 grams, %)	20	(2005)
Women 20–24 years old who gave birth before age 18 (%)	22	(2011)

WATER AND SANITATION

Improved drinking water coverage
Percentage of population, by type of drinking water source, 1990–2010

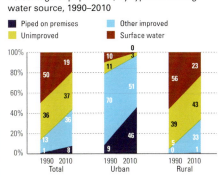

Legend: Piped on premises, Other improved, Unimproved, Surface water

Total 1990: Surface water 19, Other improved 50, Unimproved 37, Piped 36, ...13, 8
Total 2010: ...
Urban 1990: 0, 10, 11, 70, 9
Urban 2010: 3, 51, 46
Rural 1990: 23, 56, 39, 5
Rural 2010: 43, 33, 1

Source: WHO/UNICEF JMP, 2012.

Improved sanitation coverage
Percentage of population, by type of sanitation facility, 1990–2010

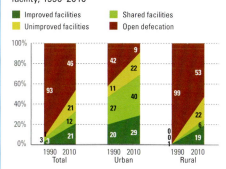

Legend: Improved facilities, Shared facilities, Unimproved facilities, Open defecation

Total 1990: 93, 12, 21, 3, 3
Total 2010: 46, 11, 27, 20, 21
Urban 1990: 42, 22, 40, 29
Urban 2010: 9, ...
Rural 1990: 99, 0, 0, 1
Rural 2010: 53, 22, 6, 19

Source: WHO/UNICEF JMP, 2012.

DISPARITIES IN NUTRITION

Indicator	Gender			Residence			Wealth quintile						Equity chart	Source
	Male	Female	Ratio of male to female	Urban	Rural	Ratio of urban to rural	Poorest	Second	Middle	Fourth	Richest	Ratio of richest to poorest		
Stunting prevalence (%)	46	43	1.1	32	46	0.7	49	48	46	45	30	0.6	▪▪▪▪▫	DHS, 2011
Underweight prevalence (%)	31	27	1.1	16	30	0.5	36	33	29	26	15	0.4	▪▪▪▪▫	DHS, 2011
Wasting prevalence (%)	11	8	1.4	6	10	0.6	12	12	9	8	5	0.4	▫▫▫▫▫	DHS, 2011
Women with low BMI (<18.5 kg/m², %)	–	27	–	20	29	0.7	32	31	27	29	19	0.6	▪▪▪▪▫	DHS, 2011
Women with high BMI (≥25 kg/m², %)	–	6	–	15	3	5.7	2	2	2	3	16	8.6	▫▫▫▫▪	DHS, 2011

GUATEMALA

Total population (000)	**14,757**	(2011)
Total under-five population (000)	**2,192**	(2011)
Total number of births (000)	**473**	(2011)
Under-five mortality rate (per 1,000 live births)	**30**	(2011)
Total number of under-five deaths (000)	**14**	(2011)
Infant mortality rate (per 1,000 live births)	**24**	(2011)
Neonatal mortality rate (per 1,000 live births)	**15**	(2011)
HIV prevalence rate (15–49 years old, %)	**0.8**	(2011)
Population below international poverty line of US$1.25 per day (%)	**14**	(2006)
GNI per capita (US$)	**2,870**	(2011)
Primary school net attendance ratio (% female, % male)	–	–

Causes of under-five deaths, 2010

Globally, undernutrition contributes to more than one third of child deaths

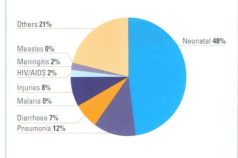

- Others 21%
- Neonatal **48%**
- Measles **0%**
- Meningitis **2%**
- HIV/AIDS **2%**
- Injuries **8%**
- Malaria **0%**
- Diarrhoea **7%**
- Pneumonia **12%**

Source: WHO/CHERG, 2012.

Under-five mortality rate

Deaths per 1,000 live births

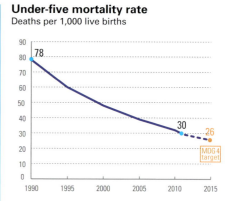

Source: IGME, 2012.

Burden of malnutrition (2011)

Stunting country rank	**25**
Share of world stunting burden (%)	**<1%**

Stunted (under-fives, 000)	**1,052**
Wasted (under-fives, 000)	**24**
Severely wasted (under-fives, 000)	**–**

MDG 1 progress	**On track**
Underweight (under-fives, 000)	**285**
Overweight (under-fives, 000)	**107**

Stunting trends

Percentage of children <5 years old stunted

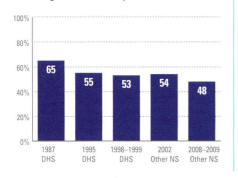

Stunting disparities

Percentage of children <5 years old stunted, by selected background characteristics

NO DATA

Underweight trends

Percentage of children <5 years old underweight

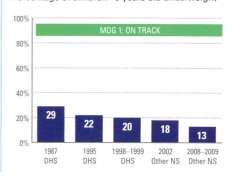

Exclusive breastfeeding trends

Percentage of infants <6 months old exclusively breastfed

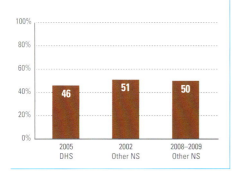

Infant feeding practices, by age

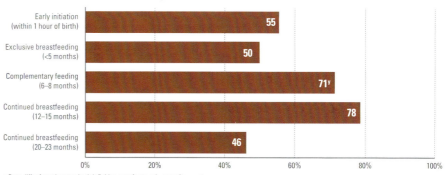

- Early initiation (within 1 hour of birth): 55
- Exclusive breastfeeding (<5 months): 50
- Complementary feeding (6–8 months): 71ʸ
- Continued breastfeeding (12–15 months): 78
- Continued breastfeeding (20–23 months): 46

y Data differ from the standard definition or refer to only part of a country.
Source: Other NS, 2008–2009.

GUATEMALA

ESSENTIAL NUTRITION PRACTICES AND INTERVENTIONS DURING THE LIFE CYCLE

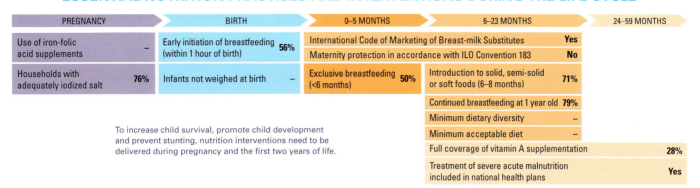

PREGNANCY	BIRTH	0–5 MONTHS	6–23 MONTHS	24–59 MONTHS

Use of iron-folic acid supplements	–	
Households with adequately iodized salt	76%	

Early initiation of breastfeeding (within 1 hour of birth)	56%	
Infants not weighed at birth	–	

International Code of Marketing of Breast-milk Substitutes	Yes
Maternity protection in accordance with ILO Convention 183	No
Exclusive breastfeeding (<6 months)	50%

Introduction to solid, semi-solid or soft foods (6–8 months)	71%
Continued breastfeeding at 1 year old	79%
Minimum dietary diversity	–
Minimum acceptable diet	–
Full coverage of vitamin A supplementation	28%
Treatment of severe acute malnutrition included in national health plans	Yes

To increase child survival, promote child development and prevent stunting, nutrition interventions need to be delivered during pregnancy and the first two years of life.

MICRONUTRIENTS

Anaemia
Prevalence of anaemia among selected populations

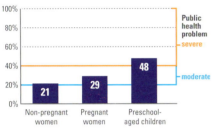

Source: Other NS, 2008–2009.

Iodized salt trends*
Percentage of households with adequately iodized salt
114,000 newborns are unprotected against iodine deficiency disorders (2011)

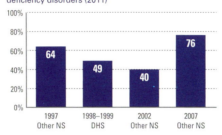

* Estimates may not be comparable.

Vitamin A supplementation
Percentage of children 6–59 months old receiving two doses of vitamin A during calendar year (full coverage)

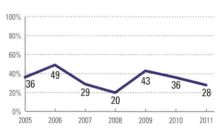

Source: UNICEF, 2012.

MATERNAL NUTRITION AND HEALTH

Maternal mortality ratio, adjusted (per 100,000 live births)	120	(2010)
Maternal mortality ratio, reported (per 100,000 live births)	140	(2007)
Total number of maternal deaths	550	(2010)
Lifetime risk of maternal death (1 in :)	190	(2010)
Women with low BMI (<18.5 kg/m², %)	2	(2008–2009)
Anaemia, non-pregnant women (<120g/l, %)	21	(2008–2009)
Antenatal care (at least one visit, %)	93	(2009)
Antenatal care (at least four visits, %)	–	–
Skilled attendant at birth (%)	52	(2009)
Low birthweight (<2,500 grams, %)	11	(2008–2009)
Women 20–24 years old who gave birth before age 18 (%)	22	(2009)

WATER AND SANITATION

Improved drinking water coverage
Percentage of population, by type of drinking water source, 1990–2010

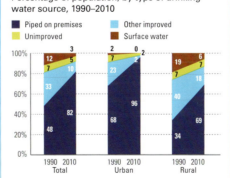

Source: WHO/UNICEF JMP, 2012.

Improved sanitation coverage
Percentage of population, by type of sanitation facility, 1990–2010

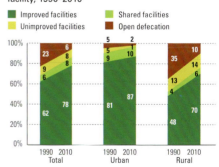

Source: WHO/UNICEF JMP, 2012.

DISPARITIES IN NUTRITION

Indicator	Gender			Residence			Wealth quintile							Source
	Male	Female	Ratio of male to female	Urban	Rural	Ratio of urban to rural	Poorest	Second	Middle	Fourth	Richest	Ratio of richest to poorest	Equity chart	
Stunting prevalence (%)	–	–	–	–	–	–	–	–	–	–	–	–		Other NS, 2008–2009
Underweight prevalence (%)	14	12	1.1	8	16	0.5	21	14	11	5	3	0.2		Other NS, 2008–2009
Wasting prevalence (%)	1	1	1.0	1	2	0.6	1	1	2	1	1	0.5		Other NS, 2008–2009
Women with low BMI (<18.5 kg/m², %)	–	2	–	2	2	1.2	1	1	1	1	3	2.1		Other NS, 2008–2009
Women with high BMI (≥25 kg/m², %)	–	51	–	58	46	1.3	37	48	55	61	61	1.7		Other NS, 2008–2009

GUINEA

DEMOGRAPHICS AND BACKGROUND INFORMATION

Total population (000)	**10,222**	(2011)
Total under-five population (000)	**1,696**	(2011)
Total number of births (000)	**394**	(2011)
Under-five mortality rate (per 1,000 live births)	**126**	(2011)
Total number of under-five deaths (000)	**48**	(2011)
Infant mortality rate (per 1,000 live births)	**79**	(2011)
Neonatal mortality rate (per 1,000 live births)	**39**	(2011)
HIV prevalence rate (15–49 years old, %)	**1.4**	(2011)
Population below international poverty line of US$1.25 per day (%)	**43**	(2007)
GNI per capita (US$)	**440**	(2011)
Primary school net attendance ratio (% female, % male)	**48, 55**	(2005)

Causes of under-five deaths, 2010
Globally, undernutrition contributes to more than one third of child deaths

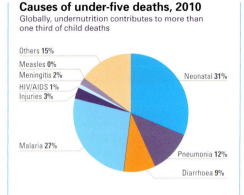

Others 15%
Measles 0%
Meningitis 2%
HIV/AIDS 1%
Injuries 3%
Neonatal 31%
Malaria 27%
Pneumonia 12%
Diarrhoea 9%

Source: WHO/CHERG, 2012.

Under-five mortality rate
Deaths per 1,000 live births

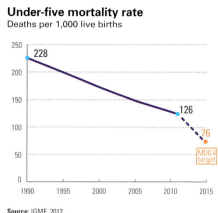

Source: IGME, 2012.

NUTRITIONAL STATUS

Burden of malnutrition (2011)

Stunting country rank	**34**
Share of world stunting burden (%)	**<1%**

Stunted (under-fives, 000)	**678**
Wasted (under-fives, 000)	**141**
Severely wasted (under-fives, 000)	**47**

MDG 1 progress	**No progress**
Underweight (under-fives, 000)	**353**
Overweight (under-fives, 000)	**–**

Stunting trends
Percentage of children <5 years old stunted

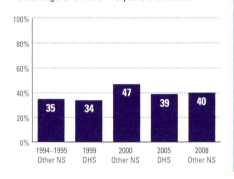

1994–1995 Other NS	1999 DHS	2000 Other NS	2005 DHS	2008 Other NS
35	34	47	39	40

Stunting disparities
Percentage of children <5 years old stunted, by selected background characteristics

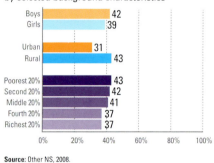

Boys 42
Girls 39
Urban 31
Rural 43
Poorest 20% 43
Second 20% 42
Middle 20% 41
Fourth 20% 37
Richest 20% 37

Source: Other NS, 2008.

Underweight trends
Percentage of children <5 years old underweight

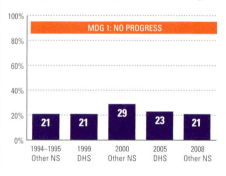

MDG 1: NO PROGRESS

1994–1995 Other NS	1999 DHS	2000 Other NS	2005 DHS	2008 Other NS
21	21	29	23	21

INFANT AND YOUNG CHILD FEEDING

Exclusive breastfeeding trends
Percentage of infants <6 months old exclusively breastfed

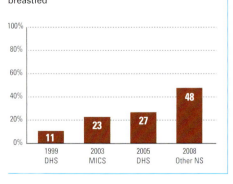

1999 DHS	2003 MICS	2005 DHS	2008 Other NS
11	23	27	48

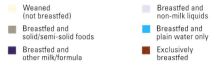

Weaned (not breastfed)
Breastfed and solid/semi-solid foods
Breastfed and other milk/formula
Breastfed and non-milk liquids
Breastfed and plain water only
Exclusively breastfed

Infant feeding practices, by age

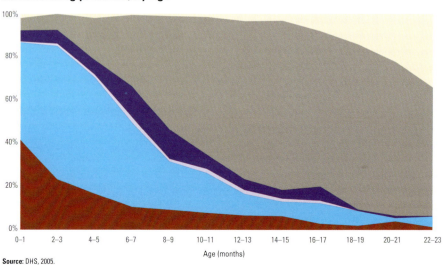

Age (months)

Source: DHS, 2005.

ESSENTIAL NUTRITION PRACTICES AND INTERVENTIONS DURING THE LIFE CYCLE

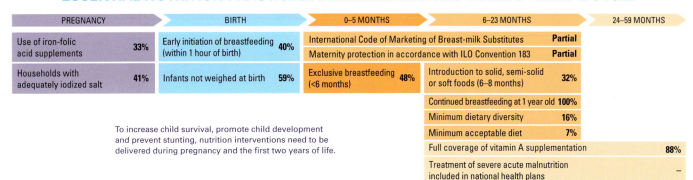

PREGNANCY	BIRTH	0–5 MONTHS	6–23 MONTHS	24–59 MONTHS

| Use of iron-folic acid supplements | 33% |
| Households with adequately iodized salt | 41% |

| Early initiation of breastfeeding (within 1 hour of birth) | 40% |
| Infants not weighed at birth | 59% |

International Code of Marketing of Breast-milk Substitutes	Partial
Maternity protection in accordance with ILO Convention 183	Partial
Exclusive breastfeeding (<6 months)	48%

Introduction to solid, semi-solid or soft foods (6–8 months)	32%
Continued breastfeeding at 1 year old	100%
Minimum dietary diversity	16%
Minimum acceptable diet	7%
Full coverage of vitamin A supplementation	88%
Treatment of severe acute malnutrition included in national health plans	–

To increase child survival, promote child development and prevent stunting, nutrition interventions need to be delivered during pregnancy and the first two years of life.

MICRONUTRIENTS

Anaemia
Prevalence of anaemia among selected populations

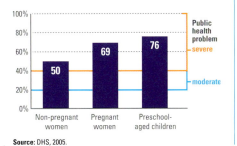

Non-pregnant women: 50
Pregnant women: 69
Preschool-aged children: 76

Public health problem — severe / moderate

Source: DHS, 2005.

Iodized salt trends*
Percentage of households with adequately iodized salt

232,000 newborns are unprotected against iodine deficiency disorders (2011)

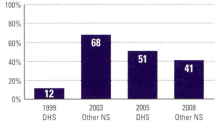

1999 DHS	2003 Other NS	2005 DHS	2008 Other NS
12	68	51	41

* Estimates may not be comparable.

Vitamin A supplementation
Percentage of children 6–59 months old receiving two doses of vitamin A during calendar year (full coverage)

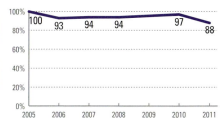

2005: 100, 2006: 93, 2007: 94, 2008: 94, 2010: 97, 2011: 88

Source: UNICEF, 2012.

MATERNAL NUTRITION AND HEALTH

Maternal mortality ratio, adjusted (per 100,000 live births)	610	(2010)
Maternal mortality ratio, reported (per 100,000 live births)	980	(2005)
Total number of maternal deaths	2,400	(2010)
Lifetime risk of maternal death (1 in :)	30	(2010)
Women with low BMI (<18.5 kg/m², %)	–	–
Anaemia, non-pregnant women (<120g/l, %)	50	(2005)
Antenatal care (at least one visit, %)	88	(2007)
Antenatal care (at least four visits, %)	50	(2007)
Skilled attendant at birth (%)	46	(2007)
Low birthweight (<2,500 grams, %)	12	(2005)
Women 20–24 years old who gave birth before age 18 (%)	44	(2005)

WATER AND SANITATION

Improved drinking water coverage
Percentage of population, by type of drinking water source, 1990–2010

Piped on premises / Other improved / Unimproved / Surface water

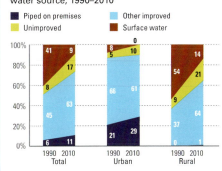

Source: WHO/UNICEF JMP, 2012.

Improved sanitation coverage
Percentage of population, by type of sanitation facility, 1990–2010

Improved facilities / Shared facilities / Unimproved facilities / Open defecation

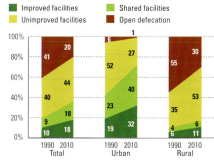

Source: WHO/UNICEF JMP, 2012.

DISPARITIES IN NUTRITION

Indicator	Gender			Residence			Wealth quintile						Equity chart	Source
	Male	Female	Ratio of male to female	Urban	Rural	Ratio of urban to rural	Poorest	Second	Middle	Fourth	Richest	Ratio of richest to poorest		
Stunting prevalence (%)	42	39	1.1	31	43	0.7	43	42	41	37	37	0.9	▪▪▪▪▪	Other NS, 2008
Underweight prevalence (%)	22	20	1.1	15	23	0.7	24	22	21	19	19	0.8	▪▪▪▪▪	Other NS, 2008
Wasting prevalence (%)	9	8	1.1	8	9	0.9	–	–	–	–	–	–		Other NS, 2008
Women with low BMI (<18.5 kg/m², %)	–	–	–	–	–	–	–	–	–	–	–	–		–
Women with high BMI (≥25 kg/m², %)	–	–	–	–	–	–	–	–	–	–	–	–		–

INDIA

DEMOGRAPHICS AND BACKGROUND INFORMATION

Total population (000)	1,241,492	(2011)
Total under-five population (000)	128,589	(2011)
Total number of births (000)	27,098	(2011)
Under-five mortality rate (per 1,000 live births)	61	(2011)
Total number of under-five deaths (000)	1,655	(2011)
Infant mortality rate (per 1,000 live births)	47	(2011)
Neonatal mortality rate (per 1,000 live births)	32	(2011)
HIV prevalence rate (15–49 years old, %)	–	–
Population below international poverty line of US$1.25 per day (%)	33	(2010)
GNI per capita (US$)	1,410	(2011)
Primary school net attendance ratio (% female, % male)	81, 85	(2005–2006)

Causes of under-five deaths, 2010
Globally, undernutrition contributes to more than one third of child deaths

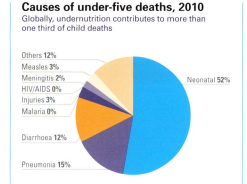

Others **12%**
Measles **3%**
Meningitis **2%**
HIV/AIDS **0%**
Injuries **3%**
Malaria **0%**
Diarrhoea **12%**
Pneumonia **15%**
Neonatal **52%**

Source: WHO/CHERG, 2012.

Under-five mortality rate
Deaths per 1,000 live births

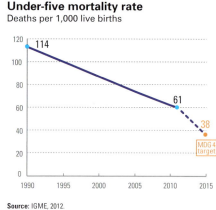

Source: IGME, 2012.

NUTRITIONAL STATUS

Burden of malnutrition (2011)

Stunting country rank	1
Share of world stunting burden (%)	38

Stunted (under-fives, 000)	61,723	MDG 1 progress	**Insufficient progress**
Wasted (under-fives, 000)	25,461	Underweight (under-fives, 000)	54,650
Severely wasted (under-fives, 000)	8,230	Overweight (under-fives, 000)	2,443

Stunting trends
Percentage of children <5 years old stunted

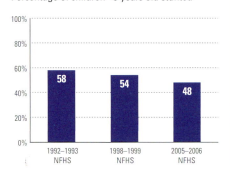

1992–1993 NFHS	1998–1999 NFHS	2005–2006 NFHS
58	54	48

Stunting disparities
Percentage of children <5 years old stunted, by selected background characteristics

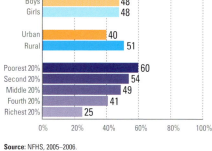

Boys 48
Girls 48
Urban 40
Rural 51
Poorest 20% 60
Second 20% 54
Middle 20% 49
Fourth 20% 41
Richest 20% 25

Source: NFHS, 2005–2006.

Underweight trends
Percentage of children <5 years old underweight

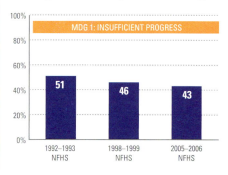

MDG 1: INSUFFICIENT PROGRESS

1992–1993 NFHS	1998–1999 NFHS	2005–2006 NFHS
51	46	43

INFANT AND YOUNG CHILD FEEDING

Exclusive breastfeeding trends
Percentage of infants <6 months old exclusively breastfed

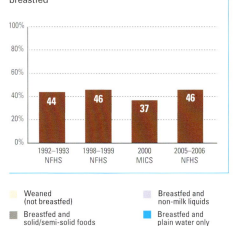

1992–1993 NFHS	1998–1999 NFHS	2000 MICS	2005–2006 NFHS
44	46	37	46

Infant feeding practices, by age

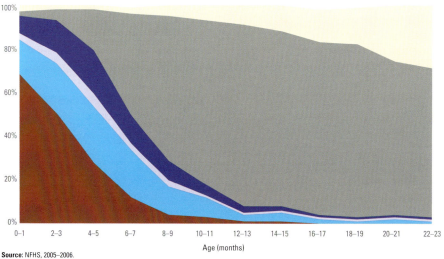

Weaned (not breastfed)
Breastfed and solid/semi-solid foods
Breastfed and other milk/formula
Breastfed and non-milk liquids
Breastfed and plain water only
Exclusively breastfed

Source: NFHS, 2005–2006.

INDIA

ESSENTIAL NUTRITION PRACTICES AND INTERVENTIONS DURING THE LIFE CYCLE

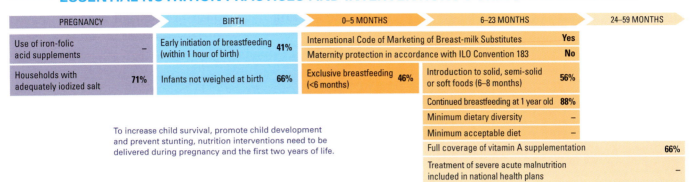

PREGNANCY	BIRTH	0–5 MONTHS	6–23 MONTHS	24–59 MONTHS

Use of iron-folic acid supplements	–	Early initiation of breastfeeding (within 1 hour of birth)	41%	International Code of Marketing of Breast-milk Substitutes	Yes
				Maternity protection in accordance with ILO Convention 183	No
Households with adequately iodized salt	71%	Infants not weighed at birth	66%	Exclusive breastfeeding (<6 months)	46%

Introduction to solid, semi-solid or soft foods (6–8 months) — 56%
Continued breastfeeding at 1 year old — 88%
Minimum dietary diversity — –
Minimum acceptable diet — –
Full coverage of vitamin A supplementation — 66%
Treatment of severe acute malnutrition included in national health plans — –

To increase child survival, promote child development and prevent stunting, nutrition interventions need to be delivered during pregnancy and the first two years of life.

MICRONUTRIENTS

Anaemia
Prevalence of anaemia among selected populations

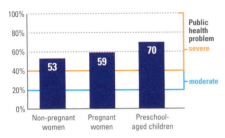

Source: NFHS, 2005–2006.

Iodized salt trends*
Percentage of households with adequately iodized salt

7,831,000 newborns are unprotected against iodine deficiency disorders (2011)

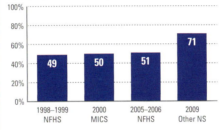

* Estimates may not be comparable.

Vitamin A supplementation
Percentage of children 6–59 months old receiving two doses of vitamin A during calendar year (full coverage)

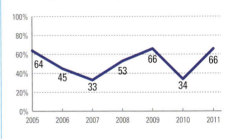

Source: UNICEF, 2012.

MATERNAL NUTRITION AND HEALTH

Maternal mortality ratio, adjusted (per 100,000 live births)	200	(2010)
Maternal mortality ratio, reported (per 100,000 live births)	210	(2009)
Total number of maternal deaths	56,000	(2010)
Lifetime risk of maternal death (1 in :)	170	(2010)
Women with low BMI (<18.5 kg/m², %)	36	(2005–2006)
Anaemia, non-pregnant women (<120g/l, %)	53	(2005–2006)
Antenatal care (at least one visit, %)	74	(2006)
Antenatal care (at least four visits, %)	37	(2006)
Skilled attendant at birth (%)	52	(2008)
Low birthweight (<2,500 grams, %)	28	(2005–2006)
Women 20–24 years old who gave birth before age 18 (%)	22	(2006)

WATER AND SANITATION

Improved drinking water coverage
Percentage of population, by type of drinking water source, 1990–2010

Piped on premises · Other improved · Unimproved · Surface water

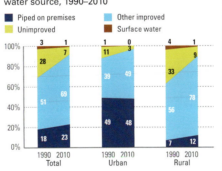

Source: WHO/UNICEF JMP, 2012.

Improved sanitation coverage
Percentage of population, by type of sanitation facility, 1990–2010

Improved facilities · Shared facilities · Unimproved facilities · Open defecation

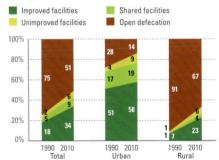

Source: WHO/UNICEF JMP, 2012.

DISPARITIES IN NUTRITION

Indicator	Gender			Residence			Wealth quintile							Source
	Male	Female	Ratio of male to female	Urban	Rural	Ratio of urban to rural	Poorest	Second	Middle	Fourth	Richest	Ratio of richest to poorest	Equity chart	
Stunting prevalence (%)	48	48	1.0	40	51	0.8	60	54	49	41	25	0.4		NFHS, 2005–2006
Underweight prevalence (%)	42	43	1.0	33	46	0.7	57	49	41	34	20	0.3		NFHS, 2005–2006
Wasting prevalence (%)	21	19	1.1	17	21	0.8	25	22	19	17	13	0.5		NFHS, 2005–2006
Women with low BMI (<18.5 kg/m², %)	–	36	–	25	41	0.6	52	46	38	29	18	0.4		NFHS, 2005–2006
Women with high BMI (≥25 kg/m², %)	–	13	–	24	7	3.2	2	4	7	15	31	16.9		NFHS, 2005–2006

INDONESIA

Total population (000)	**242,326**	(2011)
Total under-five population (000)	**21,199**	(2011)
Total number of births (000)	**4,331**	(2011)
Under-five mortality rate (per 1,000 live births)	**32**	(2011)
Total number of under-five deaths (000)	**134**	(2011)
Infant mortality rate (per 1,000 live births)	**25**	(2011)
Neonatal mortality rate (per 1,000 live births)	**15**	(2011)
HIV prevalence rate (15–49 years old, %)	**0.3**	(2011)
Population below international poverty line of US$1.25 per day (%)	**18**	(2010)
GNI per capita (US$)	**2,940**	(2011)
Primary school net attendance ratio (% female, % male)	**98, 98**	(2010)

Causes of under-five deaths, 2010
Globally, undernutrition contributes to more than one third of child deaths

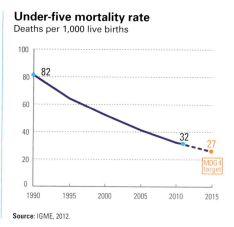

Others **20%**
Neonatal **48%**
Measles **5%**
Meningitis **2%**
HIV/AIDS **0%**
Injuries **6%**
Malaria **2%**
Diarrhoea **5%**
Pneumonia **12%**

Source: WHO/CHERG, 2012.

Under-five mortality rate
Deaths per 1,000 live births

82
32
27
MDG 4 target

Source: IGME, 2012.

Burden of malnutrition (2011)

Stunting country rank	5
Share of world stunting burden (%)	5

Stunted (under-fives, 000)	**7,547**
Wasted (under-fives, 000)	**2,820**
Severely wasted (under-fives, 000)	**1,272**

MDG 1 progress	**On track**
Underweight (under-fives, 000)	**3,795**
Overweight (under-fives, 000)	**2,968**

Stunting trends
Percentage of children <5 years old stunted

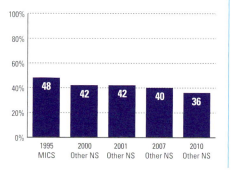

1995 MICS	2000 Other NS	2001 Other NS	2007 Other NS	2010 Other NS
48	42	42	40	36

Stunting disparities
Percentage of children <5 years old stunted, by selected background characteristics

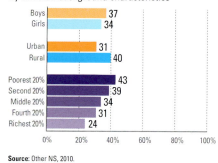

Boys 37
Girls 34
Urban 31
Rural 40
Poorest 20% 43
Second 20% 39
Middle 20% 34
Fourth 20% 31
Richest 20% 24

Source: Other NS, 2010.

Underweight trends
Percentage of children <5 years old underweight

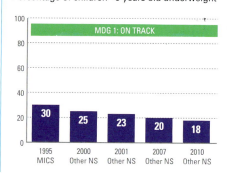

MDG 1: ON TRACK

1995 MICS	2000 Other NS	2001 Other NS	2007 Other NS	2010 Other NS
30	25	23	20	18

Exclusive breastfeeding trends
Percentage of infants <6 months old exclusively breastfed

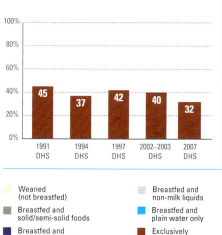

1991 DHS	1994 DHS	1997 DHS	2002–2003 DHS	2007 DHS
45	37	42	40	32

Weaned (not breastfed)
Breastfed and solid/semi-solid foods
Breastfed and other milk/formula
Breastfed and non-milk liquids
Breastfed and plain water only
Exclusively breastfed

Infant feeding practices, by age

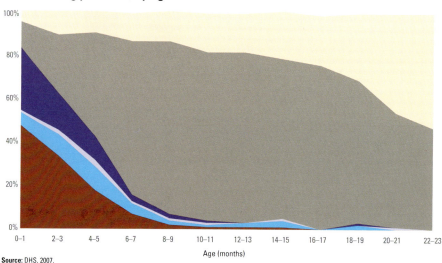

Age (months)

Source: DHS, 2007.

INDONESIA

ESSENTIAL NUTRITION PRACTICES AND INTERVENTIONS DURING THE LIFE CYCLE

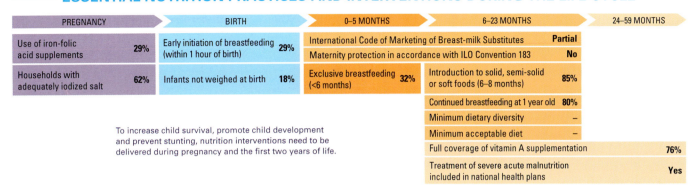

PREGNANCY	BIRTH	0–5 MONTHS	6–23 MONTHS	24–59 MONTHS

Use of iron-folic acid supplements	29%	
Households with adequately iodized salt	62%	

Early initiation of breastfeeding (within 1 hour of birth)	29%
Infants not weighed at birth	18%

International Code of Marketing of Breast-milk Substitutes	Partial
Maternity protection in accordance with ILO Convention 183	No
Exclusive breastfeeding (<6 months)	32%

Introduction to solid, semi-solid or soft foods (6–8 months)	85%
Continued breastfeeding at 1 year old	80%
Minimum dietary diversity	–
Minimum acceptable diet	–
Full coverage of vitamin A supplementation	76%
Treatment of severe acute malnutrition included in national health plans	Yes

To increase child survival, promote child development and prevent stunting, nutrition interventions need to be delivered during pregnancy and the first two years of life.

MICRONUTRIENTS

Anaemia
Prevalence of anaemia among selected populations

NO DATA

Iodized salt trends*
Percentage of households with adequately iodized salt

1,633,000 newborns are unprotected against iodine deficiency disorders (2011)

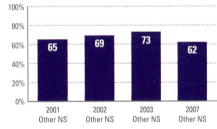

2001 Other NS	2002 Other NS	2003 Other NS	2007 Other NS
65	69	73	62

* Estimates may not be comparable.

Vitamin A supplementation
Percentage of children 6–59 months old receiving two doses of vitamin A during calendar year (full coverage)

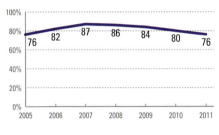

76, 82, 87, 86, 84, 80, 76 (2005–2011)

Source: UNICEF, 2012.

MATERNAL NUTRITION AND HEALTH

Maternal mortality ratio, adjusted (per 100,000 live births)	220	(2010)
Maternal mortality ratio, reported (per 100,000 live births)	230	(2007)
Total number of maternal deaths	9,600	(2010)
Lifetime risk of maternal death (1 in :)	210	(2010)
Women with low BMI (<18.5 kg/m², %)	–	–
Anaemia, non-pregnant women (<120g/l, %)	–	–
Antenatal care (at least one visit, %)	93	(2010)
Antenatal care (at least four visits, %)	82	(2007)
Skilled attendant at birth (%)	79	(2007)
Low birthweight (<2,500 grams, %)	9	(2007)
Women 20–24 years old who gave birth before age 18 (%)	10	(2007)

WATER AND SANITATION

Improved drinking water coverage
Percentage of population, by type of drinking water source, 1990–2010

Legend: Piped on premises, Other improved, Unimproved, Surface water

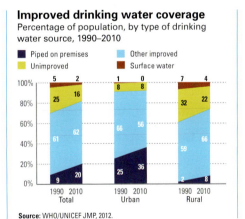

Total 1990: 5, 25, 61, 9 / 2010: 2, 16, 62, 20
Urban 1990: 1, 8, 66, 25 / 2010: 0, 8, 56, 36
Rural 1990: 7, 32, 59, 2 / 2010: 4, 22, 66, 8

Source: WHO/UNICEF JMP, 2012.

Improved sanitation coverage
Percentage of population, by type of sanitation facility, 1990–2010

Legend: Improved facilities, Shared facilities, Unimproved facilities, Open defecation

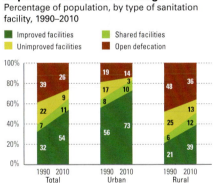

Total 1990: 39, 26, 22, 7, 32 / 2010: ...
Urban 1990: 19, 14, 9, 11, 56 / 2010: 3, 10, 73
Rural 1990: 48, 36, 13, 12, 6, 21 / 2010: 39

Source: WHO/UNICEF JMP, 2012.

DISPARITIES IN NUTRITION

Indicator	Gender			Residence			Wealth quintile						Equity chart	Source
	Male	Female	Ratio of male to female	Urban	Rural	Ratio of urban to rural	Poorest	Second	Middle	Fourth	Richest	Ratio of richest to poorest		
Stunting prevalence (%)	37	34	1.1	31	40	0.8	43	39	34	31	24	0.6	▬▬▬▬▬	Other NS, 2010
Underweight prevalence (%)	19	17	1.1	15	21	0.7	23	19	18	15	10	0.5	▬▬▬▬▬	Other NS, 2010
Wasting prevalence (%)	14	13	1.1	13	14	0.9	15	14	13	12	11	0.7	▬▬▬▬▬	Other NS, 2010
Women with low BMI (<18.5 kg/m², %)	–	–	–	–	–	–	–	–	–	–	–	–		–
Women with high BMI (≥25 kg/m², %)	–	–	–	–	–	–	–	–	–	–	–	–		–

LIBERIA

Total population (000)	**4,129**	(2011)
Total under-five population (000)	**696**	(2011)
Total number of births (000)	**157**	(2011)
Under-five mortality rate (per 1,000 live births)	**78**	(2011)
Total number of under-five deaths (000)	**12**	(2011)
Infant mortality rate (per 1,000 live births)	**58**	(2011)
Neonatal mortality rate (per 1,000 live births)	**27**	(2011)
HIV prevalence rate (15–49 years old, %)	**1.0**	(2011)
Population below international poverty line of US$1.25 per day (%)	**84**	(2007)
GNI per capita (US$)	**240**	(2011)
Primary school net attendance ratio (% female, % male)	**28, 32**	(2007)

Causes of under-five deaths, 2010
Globally, undernutrition contributes to more than one third of child deaths

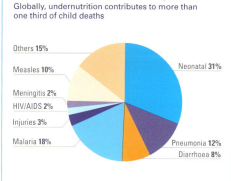

Others 15%
Measles 10%
Meningitis 2%
HIV/AIDS 2%
Injuries 3%
Malaria 18%
Neonatal 31%
Pneumonia 12%
Diarrhoea 8%

Source: WHO/CHERG, 2012.

Under-five mortality rate
Deaths per 1,000 live births

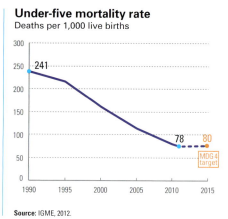

Source: IGME, 2012.

Burden of malnutrition (2011)

Stunting country rank	**49**
Share of world stunting burden (%)	**<1%**

Stunted (under-fives, 000)	**291**
Wasted (under-fives, 000)	**19**
Severely wasted (under-fives, 000)	**1**

MDG 1 progress	**On track**
Underweight (under-fives, 000)	**104**
Overweight (under-fives, 000)	**27**

Stunting trends
Percentage of children <5 years old stunted

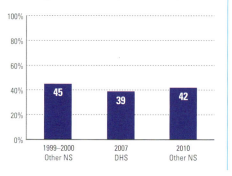

Stunting disparities
Percentage of children <5 years old stunted, by selected background characteristics

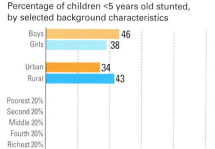

Boys 46
Girls 38
Urban 34
Rural 43
Poorest 20%
Second 20%
Middle 20%
Fourth 20%
Richest 20%

Source: Other NS, 2010.

Underweight trends
Percentage of children <5 years old underweight

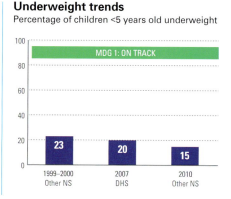

MDG 1: ON TRACK

Exclusive breastfeeding trends
Percentage of infants <6 months old exclusively breastfed

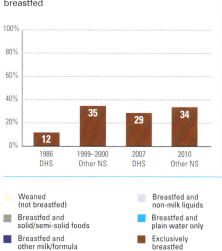

Infant feeding practices, by age

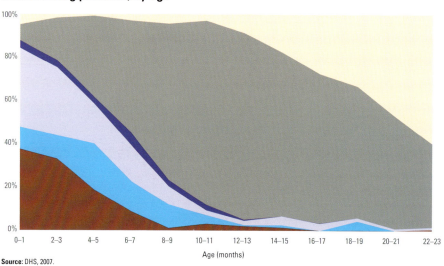

Weaned (not breastfed)
Breastfed and solid/semi-solid foods
Breastfed and other milk/formula
Breastfed and non-milk liquids
Breastfed and plain water only
Exclusively breastfed

Source: DHS, 2007.

LIBERIA

ESSENTIAL NUTRITION PRACTICES AND INTERVENTIONS DURING THE LIFE CYCLE

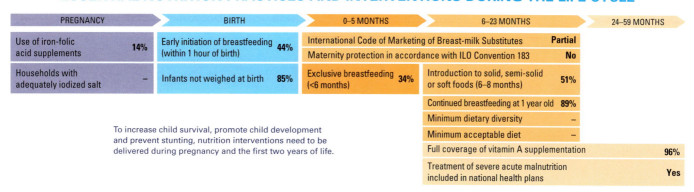

| PREGNANCY | BIRTH | 0–5 MONTHS | 6–23 MONTHS | 24–59 MONTHS |

Use of iron-folic acid supplements	**14%**	Early initiation of breastfeeding (within 1 hour of birth)	**44%**
Households with adequately iodized salt	**–**	Infants not weighed at birth	**85%**

International Code of Marketing of Breast-milk Substitutes	**Partial**
Maternity protection in accordance with ILO Convention 183	**No**

Exclusive breastfeeding (<6 months)	**34%**

Introduction to solid, semi-solid or soft foods (6–8 months)	**51%**
Continued breastfeeding at 1 year old	**89%**
Minimum dietary diversity	**–**
Minimum acceptable diet	**–**
Full coverage of vitamin A supplementation	**96%**
Treatment of severe acute malnutrition included in national health plans	**Yes**

To increase child survival, promote child development and prevent stunting, nutrition interventions need to be delivered during pregnancy and the first two years of life.

MICRONUTRIENTS

Anaemia
Prevalence of anaemia among selected populations

NO DATA

Iodized salt trends*
Percentage of households with adequately iodized salt

NO DATA

Vitamin A supplementation
Percentage of children 6–59 months old receiving two doses of vitamin A during calendar year (full coverage)

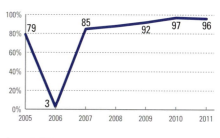

Source: UNICEF, 2012.

MATERNAL NUTRITION AND HEALTH

Maternal mortality ratio, adjusted (per 100,000 live births)	**770**	(2010)
Maternal mortality ratio, reported (per 100,000 live births)	**990**	(2007)
Total number of maternal deaths	**1,200**	(2010)
Lifetime risk of maternal death (1 in :)	**24**	(2010)
Women with low BMI (<18.5 kg/m², %)	**8**	(2010)
Anaemia, non-pregnant women (<120g/l, %)	**–**	**–**
Antenatal care (at least one visit, %)	**79**	(2007)
Antenatal care (at least four visits, %)	**66**	(2007)
Skilled attendant at birth (%)	**46**	(2007)
Low birthweight (<2,500 grams, %)	**14**	(2007)
Women 20–24 years old who gave birth before age 18 (%)	**38**	(2009)

WATER AND SANITATION

Improved drinking water coverage
Percentage of population, by type of drinking water source, 2010*

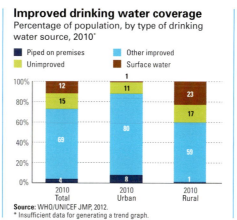

- Piped on premises
- Unimproved
- Other improved
- Surface water

Source: WHO/UNICEF JMP, 2012.
* Insufficient data for generating a trend graph.

Improved sanitation coverage
Percentage of population, by type of sanitation facility, 2010*

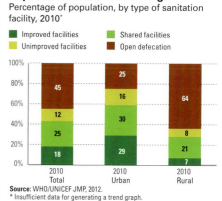

- Improved facilities
- Unimproved facilities
- Shared facilities
- Open defecation

Source: WHO/UNICEF JMP, 2012.
* Insufficient data for generating a trend graph.

DISPARITIES IN NUTRITION

Indicator	Gender			Residence			Wealth quintile						Equity chart	Source
	Male	Female	Ratio of male to female	Urban	Rural	Ratio of urban to rural	Poorest	Second	Middle	Fourth	Richest	Ratio of richest to poorest		
Stunting prevalence (%)	46	38	1.2	34	43	0.8	–	–	–	–	–	–		Other NS, 2010
Underweight prevalence (%)	17	13	1.3	–	–	–	–	–	–	–	–	–		Other NS, 2 010
Wasting prevalence (%)	8	7	1.0	9	7	1.3	7	8	10	5	8	1.1	_ _ _ _ _	Other NS, 2010
Women with low BMI (<18.5 kg/m², %)	–	8	–	–	–	–	–	–	–	–	–	–		Other NS, 2010
Women with high BMI (≥25 kg/m², %)	–	20	–	–	–	–	–	–	–	–	–	–		Other NS, 2010

MADAGASCAR

Total population (000)	21,315	(2011)
Total under-five population (000)	3,379	(2011)
Total number of births (000)	747	(2011)
Under-five mortality rate (per 1,000 live births)	62	(2011)
Total number of under-five deaths (000)	45	(2011)
Infant mortality rate (per 1,000 live births)	43	(2011)
Neonatal mortality rate (per 1,000 live births)	23	(2011)
HIV prevalence rate (15–49 years old, %)	0.3	(2011)
Population below international poverty line of US$1.25 per day (%)	81	(2010)
GNI per capita (US$)	430	(2011)
Primary school net attendance ratio (% female, % male)	80, 78	(2008–2009)

Causes of under-five deaths, 2010
Globally, undernutrition contributes to more than one third of child deaths

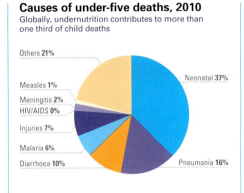

Neonatal 37%
Pneumonia 16%
Diarrhoea 10%
Malaria 6%
Injuries 7%
HIV/AIDS 0%
Meningitis 2%
Measles 1%
Others 21%

Source: WHO/CHERG, 2012.

Under-five mortality rate
Deaths per 1,000 live births

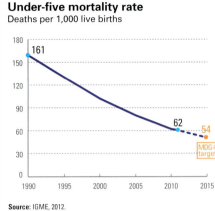

Source: IGME, 2012.

Burden of malnutrition (2011)

Stunting country rank	15
Share of world stunting burden (%)	1

Stunted (under-fives, 000)	1,693	MDG 1 progress	**No progress**
Wasted (under-fives, 000)	–	Underweight (under-fives, 000)	1,216
Severely wasted (under-fives, 000)	–	Overweight (under-fives, 000)	–

Stunting trends
Percentage of children <5 years old stunted

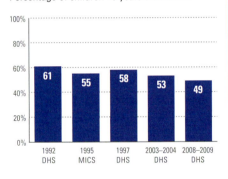

1992 DHS	1995 MICS	1997 DHS	2003–2004 DHS	2008–2009 DHS
61	55	58	53	49

Stunting disparities
Percentage of children <5 years old stunted, by selected background characteristics

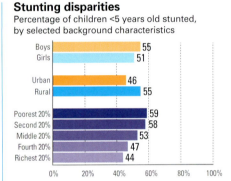

Boys	55
Girls	51
Urban	46
Rural	55
Poorest 20%	59
Second 20%	58
Middle 20%	53
Fourth 20%	47
Richest 20%	44

Source: DHS, 2003–2004.

Underweight trends
Percentage of children <5 years old underweight

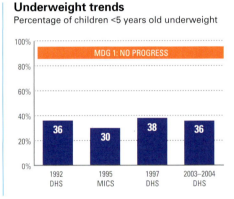

MDG 1: NO PROGRESS

1992 DHS	1995 MICS	1997 DHS	2003–2004 DHS
36	30	38	36

Exclusive breastfeeding trends
Percentage of infants <6 months old exclusively breastfed

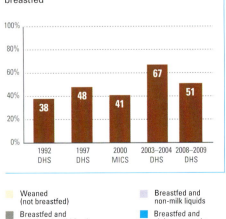

1992 DHS	1997 DHS	2000 MICS	2003–2004 DHS	2008–2009 DHS
38	48	41	67	51

Weaned (not breastfed)
Breastfed and solid/semi-solid foods
Breastfed and other milk/formula
Breastfed and non-milk liquids
Breastfed and plain water only
Exclusively breastfed

Infant feeding practices, by age

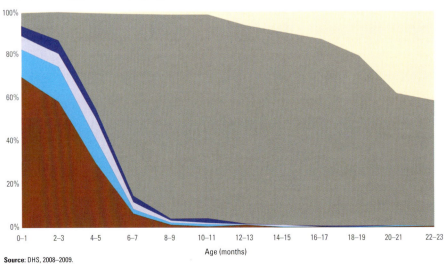

Age (months)

Source: DHS, 2008–2009.

MADAGASCAR

ESSENTIAL NUTRITION PRACTICES AND INTERVENTIONS DURING THE LIFE CYCLE

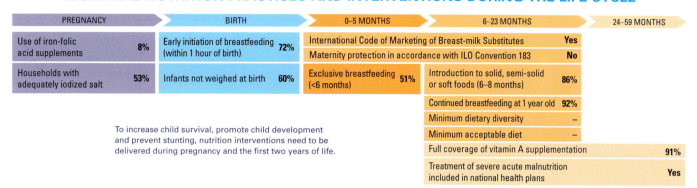

PREGNANCY	BIRTH	0–5 MONTHS	6–23 MONTHS	24–59 MONTHS

Use of iron-folic acid supplements	8%	Early initiation of breastfeeding (within 1 hour of birth)	72%
Households with adequately iodized salt	53%	Infants not weighed at birth	60%

International Code of Marketing of Breast-milk Substitutes	Yes
Maternity protection in accordance with ILO Convention 183	No
Exclusive breastfeeding (<6 months)	51%

Introduction to solid, semi-solid or soft foods (6–8 months)	86%
Continued breastfeeding at 1 year old	92%
Minimum dietary diversity	–
Minimum acceptable diet	–
Full coverage of vitamin A supplementation	91%
Treatment of severe acute malnutrition included in national health plans	Yes

To increase child survival, promote child development and prevent stunting, nutrition interventions need to be delivered during pregnancy and the first two years of life.

MICRONUTRIENTS

Anaemia
Prevalence of anaemia among selected populations

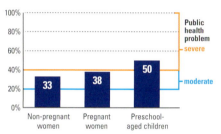

- Non-pregnant women: 33
- Pregnant women: 38
- Preschool-aged children: 50

Public health problem — severe / moderate

Source: DHS, 2008–2009.

Iodized salt trends*
Percentage of households with adequately iodized salt

354,000 newborns are unprotected against iodine deficiency disorders (2011)

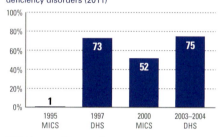

- 1995 MICS: 1
- 1997 DHS: 73
- 2000 MICS: 52
- 2003–2004 DHS: 75

* Estimates may not be comparable.

Vitamin A supplementation
Percentage of children 6–59 months old receiving two doses of vitamin A during calendar year (full coverage)

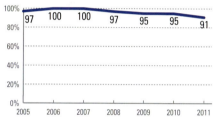

- 2005: 97
- 2006: 100
- 2007: 100
- 2008: 97
- 2009: 95
- 2010: 95
- 2011: 91

Source: UNICEF, 2012.

MATERNAL NUTRITION AND HEALTH

Maternal mortality ratio, adjusted (per 100,000 live births)	240	(2010)
Maternal mortality ratio, reported (per 100,000 live births)	500	(2009)
Total number of maternal deaths	1,800	(2010)
Lifetime risk of maternal death (1 in :)	81	(2010)
Women with low BMI (<18.5 kg/m², %)	27	(2008–2009)
Anaemia, non-pregnant women (<120g/l, %)	33	(2008–2009)
Antenatal care (at least one visit, %)	86	(2009)
Antenatal care (at least four visits, %)	49	(2009)
Skilled attendant at birth (%)	44	(2009)
Low birthweight (<2,500 grams, %)	16	(2008–2009)
Women 20–24 years old who gave birth before age 18 (%)	36	(2009)

WATER AND SANITATION

Improved drinking water coverage
Percentage of population, by type of drinking water source, 1990–2010

Legend:
- Piped on premises
- Other improved
- Unimproved
- Surface water

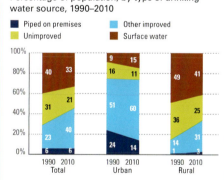

Total
- 1990: Surface water 40, Unimproved 31, Other improved 23, Piped 6
- 2010: Surface water 33, Unimproved 21, Other improved 40, Piped 6

Urban
- 1990: 9, 16, 51, 24
- 2010: 15, 11, 60, 14

Rural
- 1990: 49, 36, 14, —
- 2010: 41, 25, 31, 3

Source: WHO/UNICEF JMP, 2012.

Improved sanitation coverage
Percentage of population, by type of sanitation facility, 1990–2010

Legend:
- Improved facilities
- Shared facilities
- Unimproved facilities
- Open defecation

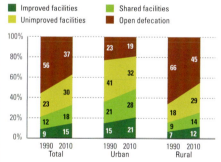

Total
- 1990: 56, 23, 12, 9
- 2010: 37, 30, 18, 15

Urban
- 1990: 23, 41, 21, 15
- 2010: 19, 32, 28, 21

Rural
- 1990: 66, 18, 9, 7
- 2010: 45, 29, 14, 12

Source: WHO/UNICEF JMP, 2012.

DISPARITIES IN NUTRITION

Indicator	Gender			Residence			Wealth quintile							Source
	Male	Female	Ratio of male to female	Urban	Rural	Ratio of urban to rural	Poorest	Second	Middle	Fourth	Richest	Ratio of richest to poorest	Equity chart	
Stunting prevalence (%)	55	51	1.1	46	55	0.8	59	58	53	47	44	0.7	▪▪▪▪▪	DHS, 2003–2004
Underweight prevalence (%)	38	33	1.1	31	37	0.8	40	41	39	29	24	0.6	▪▪▪▪–	DHS, 2003–2004
Wasting prevalence (%)	18	12	1.5	14	15	0.9	16	15	15	15	13	0.8	––––––	DHS, 2003–2004
Women with low BMI (<18.5 kg/m², %)	–	27	–	21	28	0.8	33	34	28	24	19	0.6	▪▪▪▪–	DHS, 2008–2009
Women with high BMI (≥25 kg/m², %)	–	6	–	13	5	2.7	2	2	3	6	15	8.4	–––––▪	DHS, 2008–2009

MALAWI

DEMOGRAPHICS AND BACKGROUND INFORMATION

Total population (000)	15,381	(2011)
Total under-five population (000)	2,832	(2011)
Total number of births (000)	686	(2011)
Under-five mortality rate (per 1,000 live births)	83	(2011)
Total number of under-five deaths (000)	52	(2011)
Infant mortality rate (per 1,000 live births)	53	(2011)
Neonatal mortality rate (per 1,000 live births)	27	(2011)
HIV prevalence rate (15–49 years old, %)	10.0	(2011)
Population below international poverty line of US$1.25 per day (%)	74	(2004)
GNI per capita (US$)	340	(2011)
Primary school net attendance ratio (% female, % male)	79, 76	(2006)

Causes of under-five deaths, 2010
Globally, undernutrition contributes to more than one third of child deaths

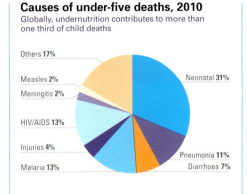

- Neonatal 31%
- Pneumonia 11%
- Diarrhoea 7%
- Malaria 13%
- Injuries 4%
- HIV/AIDS 13%
- Meningitis 2%
- Measles 2%
- Others 17%

Source: WHO/CHERG, 2012.

Under-five mortality rate
Deaths per 1,000 live births

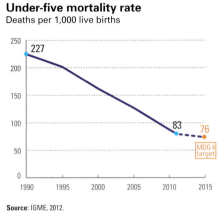

Source: IGME, 2012.

NUTRITIONAL STATUS

Burden of malnutrition (2011)

Stunting country rank	21
Share of world stunting burden (%)	<1%

Stunted (under-fives, 000)	1,334
Wasted (under-fives, 000)	113
Severely wasted (under-fives, 000)	42

MDG 1 progress	On track
Underweight (under-fives, 000)	363
Overweight (under-fives, 000)	261

Stunting trends
Percentage of children <5 years old stunted

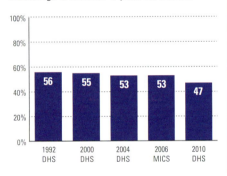

1992 DHS	2000 DHS	2004 DHS	2006 MICS	2010 DHS
56	55	53	53	47

Stunting disparities
Percentage of children <5 years old stunted, by selected background characteristics

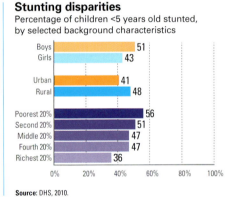

- Boys 51
- Girls 43
- Urban 41
- Rural 48
- Poorest 20% 56
- Second 20% 51
- Middle 20% 47
- Fourth 20% 47
- Richest 20% 36

Source: DHS, 2010.

Underweight trends
Percentage of children <5 years old underweight

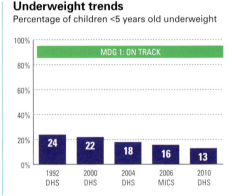

MDG 1: ON TRACK

1992 DHS	2000 DHS	2004 DHS	2006 MICS	2010 DHS
24	22	18	16	13

INFANT AND YOUNG CHILD FEEDING

Exclusive breastfeeding trends
Percentage of infants <6 months old exclusively breastfed

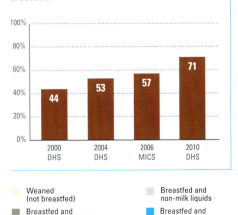

2000 DHS	2004 DHS	2006 MICS	2010 DHS
44	53	57	71

- Weaned (not breastfed)
- Breastfed and solid/semi-solid foods
- Breastfed and other milk/formula
- Breastfed and non-milk liquids
- Breastfed and plain water only
- Exclusively breastfed

Infant feeding practices, by age

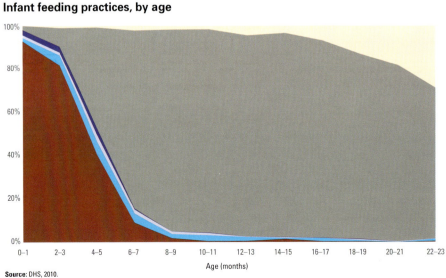

Age (months)

Source: DHS, 2010.

ESSENTIAL NUTRITION PRACTICES AND INTERVENTIONS DURING THE LIFE CYCLE

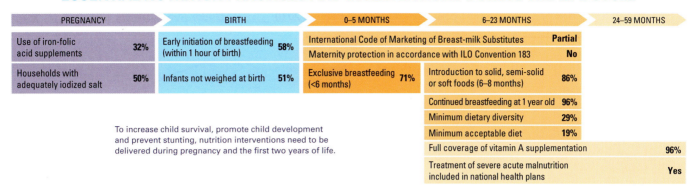

PREGNANCY	BIRTH	0–5 MONTHS	6–23 MONTHS	24–59 MONTHS

Use of iron-folic acid supplements	**32%**	Early initiation of breastfeeding (within 1 hour of birth)	**58%**	International Code of Marketing of Breast-milk Substitutes	**Partial**

International Code of Marketing of Breast-milk Substitutes	**Partial**
Maternity protection in accordance with ILO Convention 183	**No**

| Use of iron-folic acid supplements | **32%** |
| Households with adequately iodized salt | **50%** |

| Early initiation of breastfeeding (within 1 hour of birth) | **58%** |
| Infants not weighed at birth | **51%** |

| Exclusive breastfeeding (<6 months) | **71%** |

Introduction to solid, semi-solid or soft foods (6–8 months)	**86%**
Continued breastfeeding at 1 year old	**96%**
Minimum dietary diversity	**29%**
Minimum acceptable diet	**19%**

| Full coverage of vitamin A supplementation | **96%** |
| Treatment of severe acute malnutrition included in national health plans | **Yes** |

To increase child survival, promote child development and prevent stunting, nutrition interventions need to be delivered during pregnancy and the first two years of life.

MICRONUTRIENTS

Anaemia
Prevalence of anaemia among selected populations

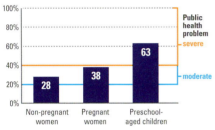

Source: DHS, 2010.

Iodized salt trends*
Percentage of households with adequately iodized salt

345,000 newborns are unprotected against iodine deficiency disorders (2011)

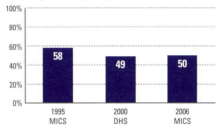

* Estimates may not be comparable.

Vitamin A supplementation
Percentage of children 6–59 months old receiving two doses of vitamin A during calendar year (full coverage)

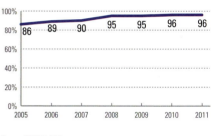

Source: UNICEF, 2012.

MATERNAL NUTRITION AND HEALTH

Maternal mortality ratio, adjusted (per 100,000 live births)	460	(2010)
Maternal mortality ratio, reported (per 100,000 live births)	680	(2010)
Total number of maternal deaths	3,000	(2010)
Lifetime risk of maternal death (1 in :)	36	(2010)
Women with low BMI (<18.5 kg/m², %)	9	(2010)
Anaemia, non-pregnant women (<120g/l, %)	28	(2010)
Antenatal care (at least one visit, %)	95	(2010)
Antenatal care (at least four visits, %)	46	(2010)
Skilled attendant at birth (%)	71	(2010)
Low birthweight (<2,500 grams, %)	13	(2006)
Women 20–24 years old who gave birth before age 18 (%)	35	(2010)

WATER AND SANITATION

Improved drinking water coverage
Percentage of population, by type of drinking water source, 1990–2010

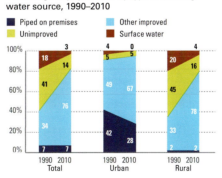

■ Piped on premises ■ Other improved
■ Unimproved ■ Surface water

Source: WHO/UNICEF JMP, 2012.

Improved sanitation coverage
Percentage of population, by type of sanitation facility, 1990–2010

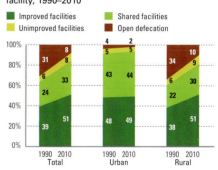

■ Improved facilities ■ Shared facilities
■ Unimproved facilities ■ Open defecation

Source: WHO/UNICEF JMP, 2012.

DISPARITIES IN NUTRITION

Indicator	Gender			Residence			Wealth quintile						Equity chart	Source
	Male	Female	Ratio of male to female	Urban	Rural	Ratio of urban to rural	Poorest	Second	Middle	Fourth	Richest	Ratio of richest to poorest		
Stunting prevalence (%)	51	43	1.2	41	48	0.8	56	51	47	47	36	0.5	■■■■■	DHS, 2010
Underweight prevalence (%)	14	12	1.2	10	13	0.8	17	14	12	14	13	0.8	– – – – –	DHS, 2010
Wasting prevalence (%)	4	4	1.1	2	4	0.6	5	5	5	4	2	0.4	– – – – –	DHS, 2010
Women with low BMI (<18.5 kg/m², %)	–	9	–	7	9	0.8	10	10	9	8	7	0.7	– – – – –	DHS, 2010
Women with high BMI (≥25 kg/m², %)	–	17	–	28	14	2.0	9	13	13	16	29	3.2	– – – – ■	DHS, 2010

MOZAMBIQUE

DEMOGRAPHICS AND BACKGROUND INFORMATION

Total population (000)	23,930	(2011)
Total under-five population (000)	3,875	(2011)
Total number of births (000)	889	(2011)
Under-five mortality rate (per 1,000 live births)	103	(2011)
Total number of under-five deaths (000)	86	(2011)
Infant mortality rate (per 1,000 live births)	72	(2011)
Neonatal mortality rate (per 1,000 live births)	34	(2011)
HIV prevalence rate (15–49 years old, %)	11.3	(2011)
Population below international poverty line of US$1.25 per day (%)	60	(2008)
GNI per capita (US$)	470	(2011)
Primary school net attendance ratio (% female, % male)	80, 82	(2008)

Causes of under-five deaths, 2010
Globally, undernutrition contributes to more than one third of child deaths

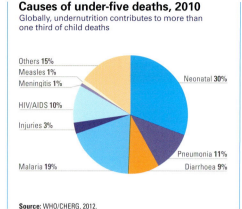

Neonatal 30%
Pneumonia 11%
Diarrhoea 9%
Malaria 19%
Injuries 3%
HIV/AIDS 10%
Meningitis 1%
Measles 1%
Others 15%

Source: WHO/CHERG, 2012.

Under-five mortality rate
Deaths per 1,000 live births

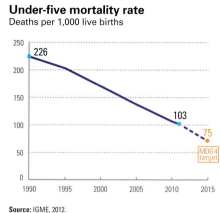

Source: IGME, 2012.

NUTRITIONAL STATUS

Burden of malnutrition (2011)

Stunting country rank	16
Share of world stunting burden (%)	1

Stunted (under-fives, 000)	1,651
Wasted (under-fives, 000)	229
Severely wasted (under-fives, 000)	81

MDG 1 progress		On track
Underweight (under-fives, 000)		577
Overweight (under-fives, 000)		287

Stunting trends
Percentage of children <5 years old stunted

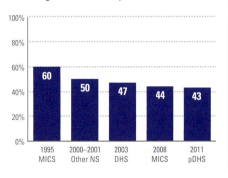

Stunting disparities
Percentage of children <5 years old stunted, by selected background characteristics

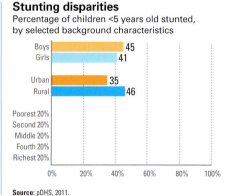

Boys 45
Girls 41
Urban 35
Rural 46
Poorest 20%
Second 20%
Middle 20%
Fourth 20%
Richest 20%

Source: pDHS, 2011.

Underweight trends
Percentage of children <5 years old underweight

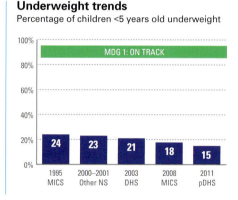

MDG 1: ON TRACK

INFANT AND YOUNG CHILD FEEDING

Exclusive breastfeeding trends
Percentage of infants <6 months old exclusively breastfed

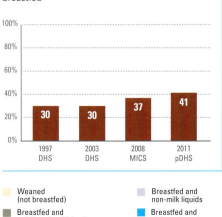

Weaned (not breastfed)

Breastfed and solid/semi-solid foods

Breastfed and other milk/formula

Breastfed and non-milk liquids

Breastfed and plain water only

Exclusively breastfed

Infant feeding practices, by age

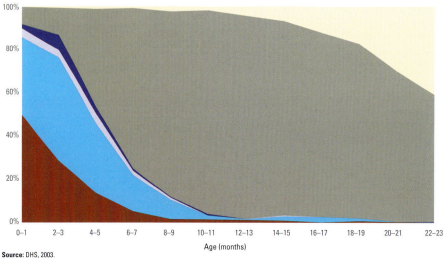

Age (months)

Source: DHS, 2003.

MOZAMBIQUE

ESSENTIAL NUTRITION PRACTICES AND INTERVENTIONS DURING THE LIFE CYCLE

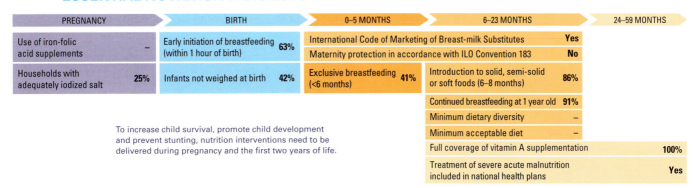

PREGNANCY	BIRTH	0–5 MONTHS	6–23 MONTHS	24–59 MONTHS

Use of iron-folic acid supplements	–	Early initiation of breastfeeding (within 1 hour of birth)	63%
Households with adequately iodized salt	25%	Infants not weighed at birth	42%

International Code of Marketing of Breast-milk Substitutes	Yes
Maternity protection in accordance with ILO Convention 183	No

Exclusive breastfeeding (<6 months)	41%

Introduction to solid, semi-solid or soft foods (6–8 months)	86%
Continued breastfeeding at 1 year old	91%
Minimum dietary diversity	–
Minimum acceptable diet	–
Full coverage of vitamin A supplementation	100%
Treatment of severe acute malnutrition included in national health plans	Yes

To increase child survival, promote child development and prevent stunting, nutrition interventions need to be delivered during pregnancy and the first two years of life.

MICRONUTRIENTS

Anaemia
Prevalence of anaemia among selected populations

NO DATA

Iodized salt trends*
Percentage of households with adequately iodized salt
666,000 newborns are unprotected against iodine deficiency disorders (2011)

1995 MICS	2003 DHS	2008 MICS
62	54	25

* Estimates may not be comparable.

Vitamin A supplementation
Percentage of children 6–59 months old receiving two doses of vitamin A during calendar year (full coverage)

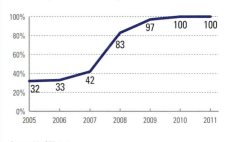

2005	2006	2007	2008	2009	2010	2011
32	33	42	83	97	100	100

Source: UNICEF, 2012.

MATERNAL NUTRITION AND HEALTH

Maternal mortality ratio, adjusted (per 100,000 live births)	490	(2010)
Maternal mortality ratio, reported (per 100,000 live births)	500	(2008)
Total number of maternal deaths	4,300	(2010)
Lifetime risk of maternal death (1 in :)	43	(2010)
Women with low BMI (<18.5 kg/m², %)	–	–
Anaemia, non-pregnant women (<120g/l, %)	–	–
Antenatal care (at least one visit, %)	92	(2008)
Antenatal care (at least four visits, %)	–	–
Skilled attendant at birth (%)	55	(2008)
Low birthweight (<2,500 grams, %)	16	(2008)
Women 20–24 years old who gave birth before age 18 (%)	42	(2003)

WATER AND SANITATION

Improved drinking water coverage
Percentage of population, by type of drinking water source, 1990–2010

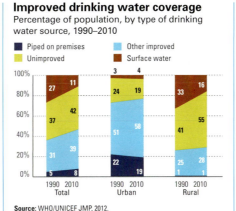

- Piped on premises
- Other improved
- Unimproved
- Surface water

Source: WHO/UNICEF JMP, 2012.

Improved sanitation coverage
Percentage of population, by type of sanitation facility, 1990–2010

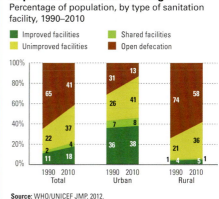

- Improved facilities
- Shared facilities
- Unimproved facilities
- Open defecation

Source: WHO/UNICEF JMP, 2012.

DISPARITIES IN NUTRITION

Indicator	Gender			Residence			Wealth quintile							Source
	Male	Female	Ratio of male to female	Urban	Rural	Ratio of urban to rural	Poorest	Second	Middle	Fourth	Richest	Ratio of richest to poorest	Equity chart	
Stunting prevalence (%)	45	41	1.1	35	46	0.8	–	–	–	–	–	–		pDHS, 2011
Underweight prevalence (%)	17	13	1.3	10	17	0.6	–	–	–	–	–	–		pDHS, 2011
Wasting prevalence (%)	6	5	1.2	4	7	0.6	–	–	–	–	–	–		pDHS, 2011
Women with low BMI (<18.5 kg/m², %)	–	–	–	–	–	–	–	–	–	–	–	–		–
Women with high BMI (≥25 kg/m², %)	–	–	–	–	–	–	–	–	–	–	–	–		–

NEPAL

Total population (000)	**30,486**	(2011)
Total under-five population (000)	**3,450**	(2011)
Total number of births (000)	**722**	(2011)
Under-five mortality rate (per 1,000 live births)	**48**	(2011)
Total number of under-five deaths (000)	**34**	(2011)
Infant mortality rate (per 1,000 live births)	**39**	(2011)
Neonatal mortality rate (per 1,000 live births)	**27**	(2011)
HIV prevalence rate (15–49 years old, %)	**0.3**	(2011)
Population below international poverty line of US$1.25 per day (%)	**25**	(2010)
GNI per capita (US$)	**540**	(2011)
Primary school net attendance ratio (% female, % male)	**70, 67**	(2010–2011)

Causes of under-five deaths, 2010
Globally, undernutrition contributes to more than one third of child deaths

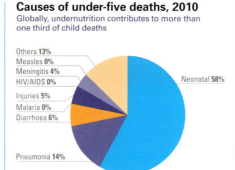

- Others **13%**
- Measles **0%**
- Meningitis **4%**
- HIV/AIDS **0%**
- Injuries **5%**
- Malaria **0%**
- Diarrhoea **6%**
- Neonatal **58%**
- Pneumonia **14%**

Source: WHO/CHERG, 2012.

Under-five mortality rate
Deaths per 1,000 live births

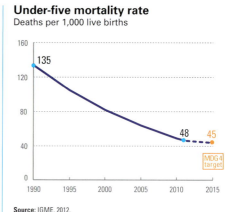

135 … 48 … 45 (MDG 4 target)

Source: IGME, 2012.

Burden of malnutrition (2011)

Stunting country rank	**20**
Share of world stunting burden (%)	**<1%**

Stunted (under-fives, 000)	**1,397**
Wasted (under-fives, 000)	**376**
Severely wasted (under-fives, 000)	**90**

MDG 1 progress	**Insufficient progress**
Underweight (under-fives, 000)	**993**
Overweight (under-fives, 000)	**48**

Stunting trends
Percentage of children <5 years old stunted

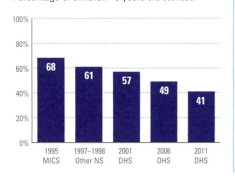

1995 MICS	1997–1998 Other NS	2001 DHS	2006 DHS	2011 DHS
68	61	57	49	41

Stunting disparities
Percentage of children <5 years old stunted, by selected background characteristics

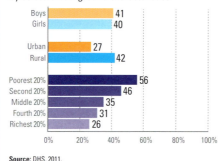

- Boys **41**
- Girls **40**
- Urban **27**
- Rural **42**
- Poorest 20% **56**
- Second 20% **46**
- Middle 20% **35**
- Fourth 20% **31**
- Richest 20% **26**

Source: DHS, 2011.

Underweight trends
Percentage of children <5 years old underweight

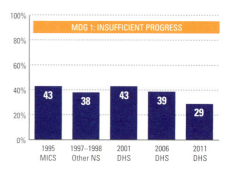

MDG 1: INSUFFICIENT PROGRESS

1995 MICS	1997–1998 Other NS	2001 DHS	2006 DHS	2011 DHS
43	38	43	39	29

Exclusive breastfeeding trends
Percentage of infants <6 months old exclusively breastfed

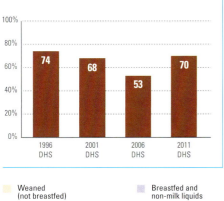

1996 DHS	2001 DHS	2006 DHS	2011 DHS
74	68	53	70

Infant feeding practices, by age

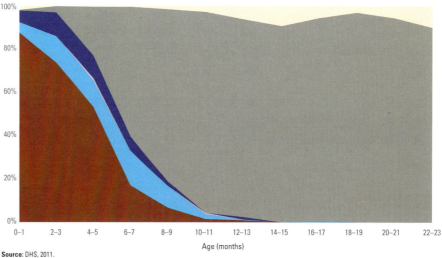

Age (months)

Source: DHS, 2011.

Legend:
- Weaned (not breastfed)
- Breastfed and solid/semi-solid foods
- Breastfed and other milk/formula
- Breastfed and non-milk liquids
- Breastfed and plain water only
- Exclusively breastfed

NEPAL

ESSENTIAL NUTRITION PRACTICES AND INTERVENTIONS DURING THE LIFE CYCLE

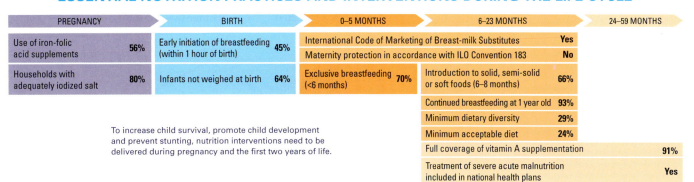

PREGNANCY	BIRTH	0–5 MONTHS	6–23 MONTHS	24–59 MONTHS

Use of iron-folic acid supplements	**56%**
Households with adequately iodized salt	**80%**

Early initiation of breastfeeding (within 1 hour of birth)	**45%**
Infants not weighed at birth	**64%**

Exclusive breastfeeding (<6 months)	**70%**

International Code of Marketing of Breast-milk Substitutes	**Yes**
Maternity protection in accordance with ILO Convention 183	**No**
Introduction to solid, semi-solid or soft foods (6–8 months)	**66%**
Continued breastfeeding at 1 year old	**93%**
Minimum dietary diversity	**29%**
Minimum acceptable diet	**24%**
Full coverage of vitamin A supplementation	**91%**
Treatment of severe acute malnutrition included in national health plans	**Yes**

To increase child survival, promote child development and prevent stunting, nutrition interventions need to be delivered during pregnancy and the first two years of life.

MICRONUTRIENTS

Anaemia
Prevalence of anaemia among selected populations

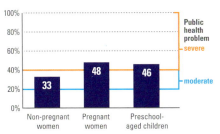

Source: DHS, 2011.

Iodized salt trends*
Percentage of households with adequately iodized salt
144,000 newborns are unprotected against iodine deficiency disorders (2011)

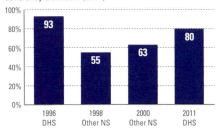

* Estimates may not be comparable.

Vitamin A supplementation
Percentage of children 6–59 months old receiving two doses of vitamin A during calendar year (full coverage)

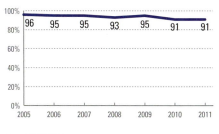

Source: UNICEF, 2012.

MATERNAL NUTRITION AND HEALTH

Maternal mortality ratio, adjusted (per 100,000 live births)	**170**	(2010)
Maternal mortality ratio, reported (per 100,000 live births)	**280**	(2005)
Total number of maternal deaths	**1,200**	(2010)
Lifetime risk of maternal death (1 in :)	**190**	(2010)
Women with low BMI (<18.5 kg/m², %)	**18**	(2011)
Anaemia, non-pregnant women (<120g/l, %)	**33**	(2011)
Antenatal care (at least one visit, %)	**58**	(2011)
Antenatal care (at least four visits, %)	**50**	(2011)
Skilled attendant at birth (%)	**36**	(2011)
Low birthweight (<2,500 grams, %)	**18**	(2011)
Women 20–24 years old who gave birth before age 18 (%)	**19**	(2011)

WATER AND SANITATION

Improved drinking water coverage
Percentage of population, by type of drinking water source, 1990–2010

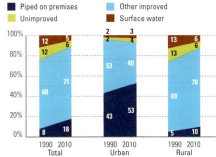

Source: WHO/UNICEF JMP, 2012.

Improved sanitation coverage
Percentage of population, by type of sanitation facility, 1990–2010

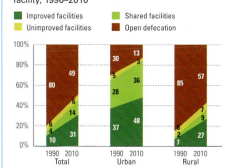

Source: WHO/UNICEF JMP, 2012.

DISPARITIES IN NUTRITION

Indicator	Gender			Residence			Wealth quintile							Source
	Male	Female	Ratio of male to female	Urban	Rural	Ratio of urban to rural	Poorest	Second	Middle	Fourth	Richest	Ratio of richest to poorest	Equity chart	
Stunting prevalence (%)	41	40	1.0	27	42	0.6	56	46	35	31	26	0.5		DHS, 2011
Underweight prevalence (%)	30	28	1.1	17	30	0.6	40	32	29	23	10	0.3		DHS, 2011
Wasting prevalence (%)	12	10	1.2	8	11	0.7	13	11	13	9	7	0.6		DHS, 2011
Women with low BMI (<18.5 kg/m², %)	–	18	–	14	19	0.8	22	21	22	17	12	0.6		DHS, 2011
Women with high BMI (≥25 kg/m², %)	–	14	–	26	11	2.3	3	6	9	15	30	9.8		DHS, 2011

NIGER

Total population (000)	**16,069**	(2011)
Total under-five population (000)	**3,200**	(2011)
Total number of births (000)	**777**	(2011)
Under-five mortality rate (per 1,000 live births)	**125**	(2011)
Total number of under-five deaths (000)	**89**	(2011)
Infant mortality rate (per 1,000 live births)	**66**	(2011)
Neonatal mortality rate (per 1,000 live births)	**32**	(2011)
HIV prevalence rate (15–49 years old, %)	**0.8**	(2011)
Population below international poverty line of US$1.25 per day (%)	**44**	(2008)
GNI per capita (US$)	**360**	(2011)
Primary school net attendance ratio (% female, % male)	**31, 44**	(2006)

Causes of under-five deaths, 2010
Globally, undernutrition contributes to more than one third of child deaths

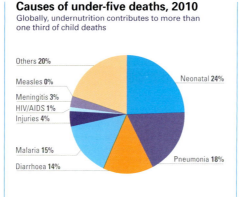

Others **20%**
Measles **0%**
Meningitis **3%**
HIV/AIDS **1%**
Injuries **4%**
Malaria **15%**
Diarrhoea **14%**
Neonatal **24%**
Pneumonia **18%**

Source: WHO/CHERG, 2012.

Under-five mortality rate
Deaths per 1,000 live births

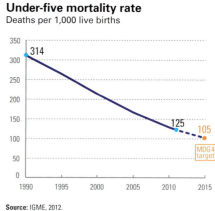

Source: IGME, 2012.

Burden of malnutrition (2011)

Stunting country rank	**18**
Share of world stunting burden (%)	**1**

Stunted (under-fives, 000)	**1,632**
Wasted (under-fives, 000)	**394**
Severely wasted (under-fives, 000)	**61**

MDG 1 progress	**No progress**
Underweight (under-fives, 000)	**1,232**
Overweight (under-fives, 000)	**112**

Stunting trends
Percentage of children <5 years old stunted

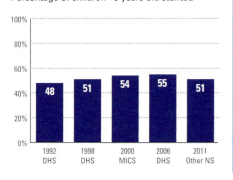

1992 DHS	1998 DHS	2000 MICS	2006 DHS	2011 Other NS
48	51	54	55	51

Stunting disparities
Percentage of children <5 years old stunted, by selected background characteristics

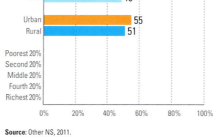

Boys **53**
Girls **49**
Urban **55**
Rural **51**
Poorest 20%
Second 20%
Middle 20%
Fourth 20%
Richest 20%

Source: Other NS, 2011.

Underweight trends
Percentage of children <5 years old underweight

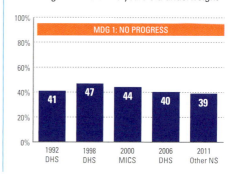

MDG 1: NO PROGRESS

1992 DHS	1998 DHS	2000 MICS	2006 DHS	2011 Other NS
41	47	44	40	39

Exclusive breastfeeding trends
Percentage of infants <6 months old exclusively breastfed

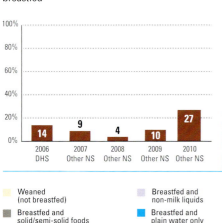

2006 DHS	2007 Other NS	2008 Other NS	2009 Other NS	2010 Other NS
14	9	4	10	27

- Weaned (not breastfed)
- Breastfed and solid/semi-solid foods
- Breastfed and other milk/formula
- Breastfed and non-milk liquids
- Breastfed and plain water only
- Exclusively breastfed

Infant feeding practices, by age

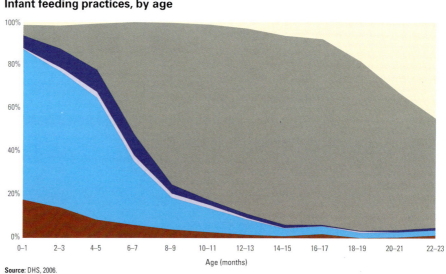

Age (months)

Source: DHS, 2006.

ESSENTIAL NUTRITION PRACTICES AND INTERVENTIONS DURING THE LIFE CYCLE

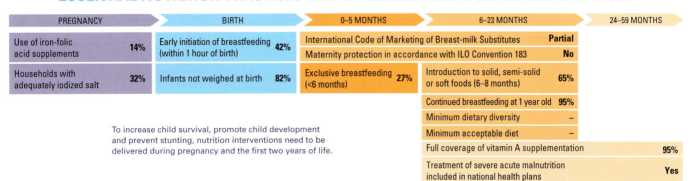

PREGNANCY	BIRTH	0–5 MONTHS	6–23 MONTHS	24–59 MONTHS

| Use of iron-folic acid supplements | 14% |
| Households with adequately iodized salt | 32% |

| Early initiation of breastfeeding (within 1 hour of birth) | 42% |
| Infants not weighed at birth | 82% |

International Code of Marketing of Breast-milk Substitutes	Partial
Maternity protection in accordance with ILO Convention 183	No
Exclusive breastfeeding (<6 months)	27%

Introduction to solid, semi-solid or soft foods (6–8 months)	65%
Continued breastfeeding at 1 year old	95%
Minimum dietary diversity	–
Minimum acceptable diet	–
Full coverage of vitamin A supplementation	95%
Treatment of severe acute malnutrition included in national health plans	Yes

To increase child survival, promote child development and prevent stunting, nutrition interventions need to be delivered during pregnancy and the first two years of life.

MICRONUTRIENTS

Anaemia
Prevalence of anaemia among selected populations

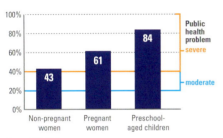

Source: DHS, 2006.

Iodized salt trends*
Percentage of households with adequately iodized salt

528,000 newborns are unprotected against iodine deficiency disorders (2011)

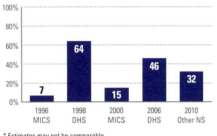

* Estimates may not be comparable.

Vitamin A supplementation
Percentage of children 6–59 months old receiving two doses of vitamin A during calendar year (full coverage)

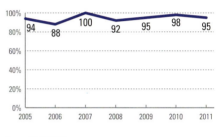

Source: UNICEF, 2012.

MATERNAL NUTRITION AND HEALTH

Maternal mortality ratio, adjusted (per 100,000 live births)	590	(2010)
Maternal mortality ratio, reported (per 100,000 live births)	650	(2006)
Total number of maternal deaths	4,500	(2010)
Lifetime risk of maternal death (1 in :)	23	(2010)
Women with low BMI (<18.5 kg/m², %)	19	(2006)
Anaemia, non-pregnant women (<120g/l, %)	43	(2006)
Antenatal care (at least one visit, %)	46	(2006)
Antenatal care (at least four visits, %)	15	(2006)
Skilled attendant at birth (%)	18	(2006)
Low birthweight (<2,500 grams, %)	27	(2006)
Women 20–24 years old who gave birth before age 18 (%)	51	(2006)

WATER AND SANITATION

Improved drinking water coverage
Percentage of population, by type of drinking water source, 1990–2010

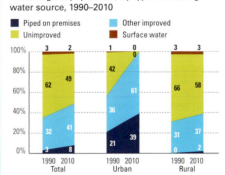

Source: WHO/UNICEF JMP, 2012.

Improved sanitation coverage
Percentage of population, by type of sanitation facility, 1990–2010

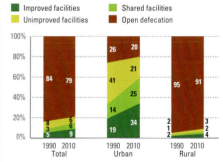

Source: WHO/UNICEF JMP, 2012.

DISPARITIES IN NUTRITION

Indicator	Gender			Residence			Wealth quintile						Equity chart	Source
	Male	Female	Ratio of male to female	Urban	Rural	Ratio of urban to rural	Poorest	Second	Middle	Fourth	Richest	Ratio of richest to poorest		
Stunting prevalence (%)	53	49	1.1	55	51	1.1	–	–	–	–	–	–		Other NS, 2011
Underweight prevalence (%)	40	37	1.1	44	39	1.1	–	–	–	–	–	–		Other NS, 2011
Wasting prevalence (%)	14	11	1.3	12	12	1.0	–	–	–	–	–	–		Other NS, 2011
Women with low BMI (<18.5 kg/m², %)	–	19	–	13	21	0.6	19	20	24	21	13	0.7		DHS, 2006
Women with high BMI (≥25 kg/m², %)	–	13	–	35	7	4.9	4	5	7	11	33	7.8		DHS, 2006

NIGERIA

Total population (000)	**162,471**	(2011)
Total under-five population (000)	**27,215**	(2011)
Total number of births (000)	**6,458**	(2011)
Under-five mortality rate (per 1,000 live births)	**124**	(2011)
Total number of under-five deaths (000)	**756**	(2011)
Infant mortality rate (per 1,000 live births)	**78**	(2011)
Neonatal mortality rate (per 1,000 live births)	**39**	(2011)
HIV prevalence rate (15–49 years old, %)	**3.7**	(2011)
Population below international poverty line of US$1.25 per day (%)	**68**	(2010)
GNI per capita (US$)	**1,200**	(2011)
Primary school net attendance ratio (% female, % male)	**60, 65**	(2008)

Causes of under-five deaths, 2010
Globally, undernutrition contributes to more than one third of child deaths

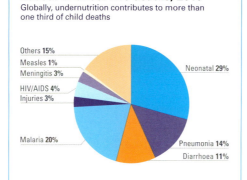

Neonatal 29%
Pneumonia 14%
Diarrhoea 11%
Malaria 20%
Injuries 3%
HIV/AIDS 4%
Meningitis 3%
Measles 1%
Others 15%

Source: WHO/CHERG, 2012.

Under-five mortality rate
Deaths per 1,000 live births

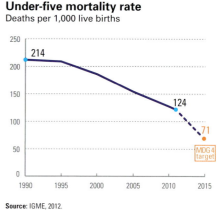

Source: IGME, 2012.

NUTRITIONAL STATUS

Burden of malnutrition (2011)

Stunting country rank	**2**
Share of world stunting burden (%)	**7**

Stunted (under-fives, 000)	**11,049**
Wasted (under-fives, 000)	**3,783**
Severely wasted (under-fives, 000)	**1,905**

MDG 1 progress	**Insufficient progress**
Underweight (under-fives, 000)	**6,287**
Overweight (under-fives, 000)	**2,858**

Stunting trends
Percentage of children <5 years old stunted

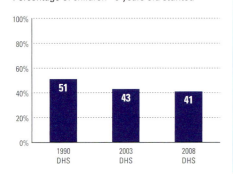

Stunting disparities
Percentage of children <5 years old stunted, by selected background characteristics

Boys 43
Girls 38
Urban 31
Rural 45
Poorest 20% 52
Second 20% 49
Middle 20% 42
Fourth 20% 34
Richest 20% 24

Source: DHS, 2008.

Underweight trends
Percentage of children <5 years old underweight

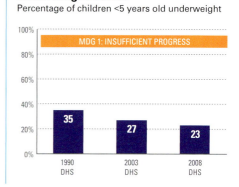

MDG 1: INSUFFICIENT PROGRESS

INFANT AND YOUNG CHILD FEEDING

Exclusive breastfeeding trends
Percentage of infants <6 months old exclusively breastfed

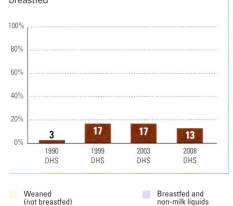

Legend:
- Weaned (not breastfed)
- Breastfed and solid/semi-solid foods
- Breastfed and other milk/formula
- Breastfed and non-milk liquids
- Breastfed and plain water only
- Exclusively breastfed

Infant feeding practices, by age

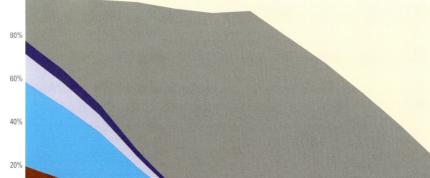

Age (months)

Source: DHS, 2008.

ESSENTIAL NUTRITION PRACTICES AND INTERVENTIONS DURING THE LIFE CYCLE

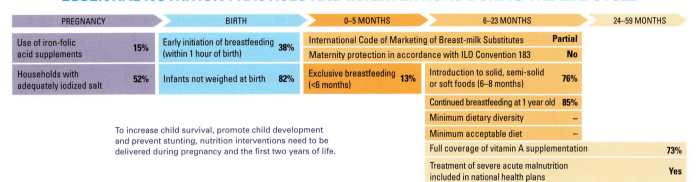

PREGNANCY	BIRTH	0–5 MONTHS	6–23 MONTHS	24–59 MONTHS

| Use of iron-folic acid supplements | 15% |
| Households with adequately iodized salt | 52% |

| Early initiation of breastfeeding (within 1 hour of birth) | 38% |
| Infants not weighed at birth | 82% |

International Code of Marketing of Breast-milk Substitutes	Partial
Maternity protection in accordance with ILO Convention 183	No
Exclusive breastfeeding (<6 months)	13%

Introduction to solid, semi-solid or soft foods (6–8 months)	76%
Continued breastfeeding at 1 year old	85%
Minimum dietary diversity	–
Minimum acceptable diet	–
Full coverage of vitamin A supplementation	73%
Treatment of severe acute malnutrition included in national health plans	Yes

To increase child survival, promote child development and prevent stunting, nutrition interventions need to be delivered during pregnancy and the first two years of life.

MICRONUTRIENTS

Anaemia
Prevalence of anaemia among selected populations

NO DATA

Iodized salt trends*
Percentage of households with adequately iodized salt

3,132,000 newborns are unprotected against iodine deficiency disorders (2011)

1998 UNICEF	98
1999 MICS	98
2003 DHS	97
2008 DHS	52

* Estimates may not be comparable.

Vitamin A supplementation
Percentage of children 6–59 months old receiving two doses of vitamin A during calendar year (full coverage)

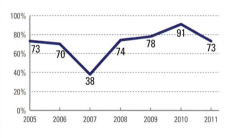

2005	2006	2007	2008	2009	2010	2011
73	70	38	74	78	91	73

Source: UNICEF, 2012.

MATERNAL NUTRITION AND HEALTH

Maternal mortality ratio, adjusted (per 100,000 live births)	630	(2010)
Maternal mortality ratio, reported (per 100,000 live births)	550	(2008)
Total number of maternal deaths	40,000	(2010)
Lifetime risk of maternal death (1 in :)	29	(2010)
Women with low BMI (<18.5 kg/m², %)	12	(2008)
Anaemia, non-pregnant women (<120g/l, %)	–	–
Antenatal care (at least one visit, %)	58	(2008)
Antenatal care (at least four visits, %)	45	(2008)
Skilled attendant at birth (%)	39	(2008)
Low birthweight (<2,500 grams, %)	12	(2008)
Women 20–24 years old who gave birth before age 18 (%)	28	(2008)

WATER AND SANITATION

Improved drinking water coverage
Percentage of population, by type of drinking water source, 1990–2010

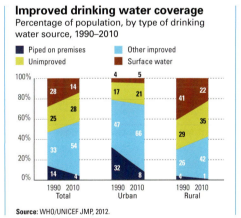

- Piped on premises
- Other improved
- Unimproved
- Surface water

Source: WHO/UNICEF JMP, 2012.

Improved sanitation coverage
Percentage of population, by type of sanitation facility, 1990–2010

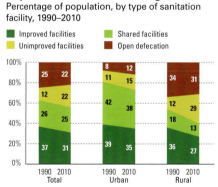

- Improved facilities
- Shared facilities
- Unimproved facilities
- Open defecation

Source: WHO/UNICEF JMP, 2012.

DISPARITIES IN NUTRITION

Indicator	Gender			Residence			Wealth quintile						Equity chart	Source
	Male	Female	Ratio of male to female	Urban	Rural	Ratio of urban to rural	Poorest	Second	Middle	Fourth	Richest	Ratio of richest to poorest		
Stunting prevalence (%)	43	38	1.1	31	45	0.7	52	49	42	34	24	0.5		DHS, 2008
Underweight prevalence (%)	25	22	1.1	16	27	0.6	35	29	22	17	10	0.3		DHS, 2008
Wasting prevalence (%)	14	13	1.1	11	15	0.7	21	17	12	10	9	0.5		DHS, 2008
Women with low BMI (<18.5 kg/m², %)	–	12	–	9	14	0.7	21	15	11	10	7	0.3		DHS, 2008
Women with high BMI (≥25 kg/m², %)	–	22	–	31	17	1.8	9	13	19	25	38	4.1		DHS, 2008

PAKISTAN

DEMOGRAPHICS AND BACKGROUND INFORMATION

Total population (000)	176,745	(2011)
Total under-five population (000)	22,113	(2011)
Total number of births (000)	4,764	(2011)
Under-five mortality rate (per 1,000 live births)	72	(2011)
Total number of under-five deaths (000)	352	(2011)
Infant mortality rate (per 1,000 live births)	59	(2011)
Neonatal mortality rate (per 1,000 live births)	36	(2011)
HIV prevalence rate (15–49 years old, %)	0.1	(2011)
Population below international poverty line of US$1.25 per day (%)	21	(2008)
GNI per capita (US$)	1,120	(2011)
Primary school net attendance ratio (% female, % male)	62, 70	(2006–2007)

Causes of under-five deaths, 2010
Globally, undernutrition contributes to more than one third of child deaths

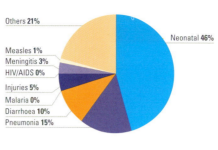

Others 21%
Neonatal 46%
Measles 1%
Meningitis 3%
HIV/AIDS 0%
Injuries 5%
Malaria 0%
Diarrhoea 10%
Pneumonia 15%

Source: WHO/CHERG, 2012.

Under-five mortality rate
Deaths per 1,000 live births

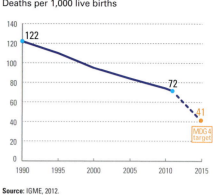

Source: IGME, 2012.

NUTRITIONAL STATUS

Burden of malnutrition (2011)

Stunting country rank	3
Share of world stunting burden (%)	6

Stunted (under-fives, 000)	9,663
Wasted (under-fives, 000)	3,339
Severely wasted (under-fives, 000)	1,283

MDG 1 progress	**Insufficient progress**
Underweight (under-fives, 000)	6,965
Overweight (under-fives, 000)	1,415

Stunting trends
Percentage of children <5 years old stunted

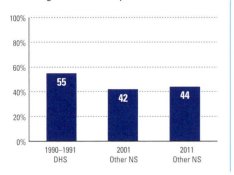

Stunting disparities
Percentage of children <5 years old stunted, by selected background characteristics

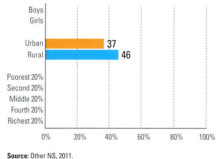

Source: Other NS, 2011.

Underweight trends
Percentage of children <5 years old underweight

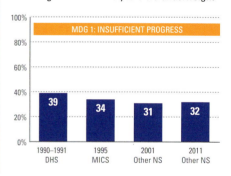

INFANT AND YOUNG CHILD FEEDING

Exclusive breastfeeding trends
Percentage of infants <6 months old exclusively breastfed

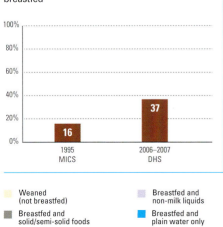

Weaned (not breastfed)

Breastfed and solid/semi-solid foods

Breastfed and other milk/formula

Breastfed and non-milk liquids

Breastfed and plain water only

Exclusively breastfed

Infant feeding practices, by age

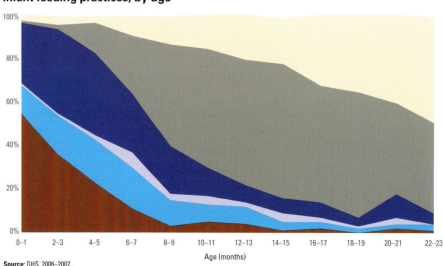

Age (months)

Source: DHS, 2006–2007.

PAKISTAN

ESSENTIAL NUTRITION PRACTICES AND INTERVENTIONS DURING THE LIFE CYCLE

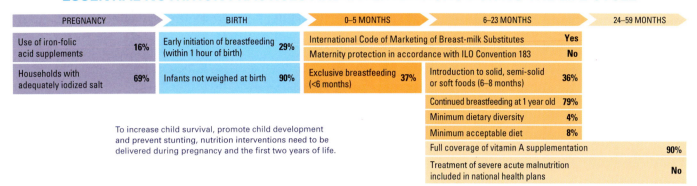

PREGNANCY	BIRTH	0–5 MONTHS	6–23 MONTHS	24–59 MONTHS

Use of iron-folic acid supplements	**16%**	Early initiation of breastfeeding (within 1 hour of birth)	**29%**	International Code of Marketing of Breast-milk Substitutes	**Yes**

Maternity protection in accordance with ILO Convention 183 — **No**

| Households with adequately iodized salt | **69%** | Infants not weighed at birth | **90%** | Exclusive breastfeeding (<6 months) | **37%** |

Introduction to solid, semi-solid or soft foods (6–8 months) — **36%**

Continued breastfeeding at 1 year old — **79%**

Minimum dietary diversity — **4%**

Minimum acceptable diet — **8%**

Full coverage of vitamin A supplementation — **90%**

Treatment of severe acute malnutrition included in national health plans — **No**

To increase child survival, promote child development and prevent stunting, nutrition interventions need to be delivered during pregnancy and the first two years of life.

MICRONUTRIENTS

Anaemia
Prevalence of anaemia among selected populations

NO DATA

Iodized salt trends*
Percentage of households with adequately iodized salt

1,467,000 newborns are unprotected against iodine deficiency disorders (2011)

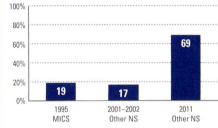

- 1995 MICS: 19
- 2001–2002 Other NS: 17
- 2011 Other NS: 69

* Estimates may not be comparable.

Vitamin A supplementation
Percentage of children 6–59 months old receiving two doses of vitamin A during calendar year (full coverage)

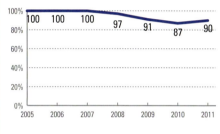

- 2005: 100
- 2006: 100
- 2007: 100
- 2008: 97
- 2009: 91
- 2010: 87
- 2011: 90

Source: UNICEF, 2012.

MATERNAL NUTRITION AND HEALTH

Maternal mortality ratio, adjusted (per 100,000 live births)	260	(2010)
Maternal mortality ratio, reported (per 100,000 live births)	280	(2007)
Total number of maternal deaths	12,000	(2010)
Lifetime risk of maternal death (1 in :)	110	(2010)
Women with low BMI (<18.5 kg/m², %)	18	(2011)
Anaemia, non-pregnant women (<120g/l, %)	–	–
Antenatal care (at least one visit, %)	61	(2007)
Antenatal care (at least four visits, %)	28	(2007)
Skilled attendant at birth (%)	43	(2011)
Low birthweight (<2,500 grams, %)	32	(2006–2007)
Women 20–24 years old who gave birth before age 18 (%)	10	(2007)

WATER AND SANITATION

Improved drinking water coverage
Percentage of population, by type of drinking water source, 1990–2010

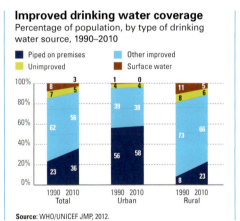

- Piped on premises
- Other improved
- Unimproved
- Surface water

Total 1990: Surface water 8, Unimproved 7, Other improved 62, Piped 23
Total 2010: Surface water 3, Unimproved 5, Other improved 56, Piped 36
Urban 1990: Surface water 1, Unimproved 4, Other improved 39, Piped 56
Urban 2010: Surface water 0, Unimproved 4, Other improved 38, Piped 58
Rural 1990: Surface water 11, Unimproved 8, Other improved 73, Piped 8
Rural 2010: Surface water 5, Unimproved 6, Other improved 66, Piped 23

Source: WHO/UNICEF JMP, 2012.

Improved sanitation coverage
Percentage of population, by type of sanitation facility, 1990–2010

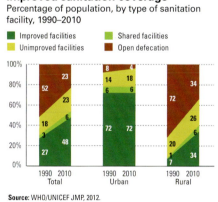

- Improved facilities
- Shared facilities
- Unimproved facilities
- Open defecation

Total 1990: Open defecation 52, Unimproved 23, Shared 6, Improved 3, 18, 27 (48)
Urban 1990: 14, 8, 6, 72
Urban 2010: 18, 4, 6, 72
Rural 1990: 72, 26, 6, 20, 1
Rural 2010: 34, 34, 7

Source: WHO/UNICEF JMP, 2012.

DISPARITIES IN NUTRITION

Indicator	Gender			Residence			Wealth quintile							Source
	Male	Female	Ratio of male to female	Urban	Rural	Ratio of urban to rural	Poorest	Second	Middle	Fourth	Richest	Ratio of richest to poorest	Equity chart	
Stunting prevalence (%)	–	–	–	37	46	0.8	–	–	–	–	–	–		Other NS, 2011
Underweight prevalence (%)	–	–	–	27	33	0.8	–	–	–	–	–	–		Other NS, 2011
Wasting prevalence (%)	–	–	–	13	16	0.8	–	–	–	–	–	–		Other NS, 2011
Women with low BMI (<18.5 kg/m², %)	–	18	–	14	20	0.7	–	–	–	–	–	–		Other NS, 2011
Women with high BMI (≥25 kg/m², %)	–	29	–	40	24	1.7	–	–	–	–	–	–		Other NS, 2011

PHILIPPINES

DEMOGRAPHICS AND BACKGROUND INFORMATION

Total population (000)	**94,852**	(2011)
Total under-five population (000)	**11,151**	(2011)
Total number of births (000)	**2,358**	(2011)
Under-five mortality rate (per 1,000 live births)	**25**	(2011)
Total number of under-five deaths (000)	**57**	(2011)
Infant mortality rate (per 1,000 live births)	**20**	(2011)
Neonatal mortality rate (per 1,000 live births)	**12**	(2011)
HIV prevalence rate (15–49 years old, %)	**<0.1**	(2011)
Population below international poverty line of US$1.25 per day (%)	**18**	(2009)
GNI per capita (US$)	**2,210**	(2011)
Primary school net attendance ratio (% female, % male)	**89, 88**	(2003)

Causes of under-five deaths, 2010
Globally, undernutrition contributes to more than one third of child deaths

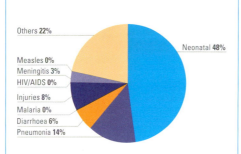

- Others **22%**
- Neonatal **48%**
- Measles **0%**
- Meningitis **3%**
- HIV/AIDS **0%**
- Injuries **8%**
- Malaria **0%**
- Diarrhoea **6%**
- Pneumonia **14%**

Source: WHO/CHERG, 2012.

Under-five mortality rate
Deaths per 1,000 live births

57 — 25 — 19 (MDG 4 target)

Source: IGME, 2012.

NUTRITIONAL STATUS

Burden of malnutrition (2011)

Stunting country rank	**9**
Share of world stunting burden (%)	**2**

Stunted (under-fives, 000)	**3,602**
Wasted (under-fives, 000)	**769**
Severely wasted (under-fives, 000)	**–**

MDG 1 progress	**Insufficient progress**
Underweight (under-fives, 000)	**2,409**
Overweight (under-fives, 000)	**368**

Stunting trends
Percentage of children <5 years old stunted

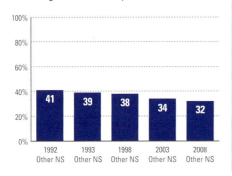

1992 Other NS	1993 Other NS	1998 Other NS	2003 Other NS	2008 Other NS
41	39	38	34	32

Stunting disparities
Percentage of children <5 years old stunted, by selected background characteristics

NO DATA

Underweight trends
Percentage of children <5 years old underweight

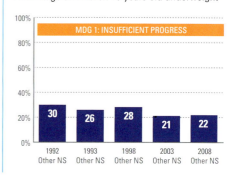

MDG 1: INSUFFICIENT PROGRESS

1992 Other NS	1993 Other NS	1998 Other NS	2003 Other NS	2008 Other NS
30	26	28	21	22

INFANT AND YOUNG CHILD FEEDING

Exclusive breastfeeding trends
Percentage of infants <6 months old exclusively breastfed

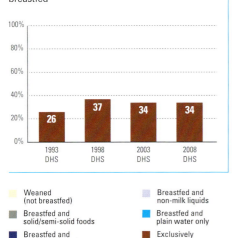

1993 DHS	1998 DHS	2003 DHS	2008 DHS
26	37	34	34

Infant feeding practices, by age

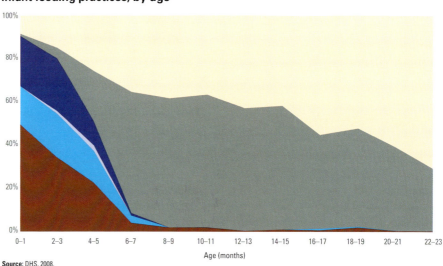

- Weaned (not breastfed)
- Breastfed and solid/semi-solid foods
- Breastfed and other milk/formula
- Breastfed and non-milk liquids
- Breastfed and plain water only
- Exclusively breastfed

Source: DHS, 2008.

PHILIPPINES

ESSENTIAL NUTRITION PRACTICES AND INTERVENTIONS DURING THE LIFE CYCLE

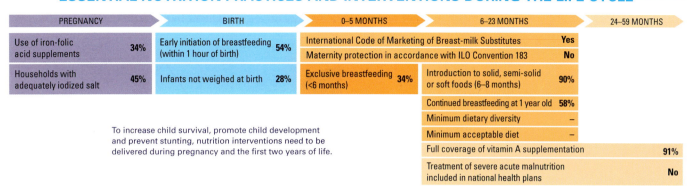

PREGNANCY	BIRTH	0–5 MONTHS	6–23 MONTHS	24–59 MONTHS

Use of iron-folic acid supplements	**34%**	Early initiation of breastfeeding (within 1 hour of birth)	**54%**	
Households with adequately iodized salt	**45%**	Infants not weighed at birth	**28%**	

International Code of Marketing of Breast-milk Substitutes	**Yes**
Maternity protection in accordance with ILO Convention 183	**No**

Exclusive breastfeeding (<6 months)	**34%**

Introduction to solid, semi-solid or soft foods (6–8 months)	**90%**
Continued breastfeeding at 1 year old	**58%**
Minimum dietary diversity	**–**
Minimum acceptable diet	**–**
Full coverage of vitamin A supplementation	**91%**
Treatment of severe acute malnutrition included in national health plans	**No**

To increase child survival, promote child development and prevent stunting, nutrition interventions need to be delivered during pregnancy and the first two years of life.

MICRONUTRIENTS

Anaemia
Prevalence of anaemia among selected populations

NO DATA

Iodized salt trends*
Percentage of households with adequately iodized salt

1,308,000 newborns are unprotected against iodine deficiency disorders (2011)

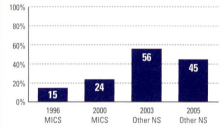

	1996 MICS	2000 MICS	2003 Other NS	2005 Other NS
	15	24	56	45

* Estimates may not be comparable.

Vitamin A supplementation
Percentage of children 6–59 months old receiving two doses of vitamin A during calendar year (full coverage)

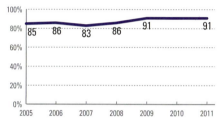

85, 86, 83, 86, 91, 91 (2005–2011)

Source: UNICEF, 2012.

MATERNAL NUTRITION AND HEALTH

Maternal mortality ratio, adjusted (per 100,000 live births)	**99**	(2010)
Maternal mortality ratio, reported (per 100,000 live births)	**160**	(2006)
Total number of maternal deaths	**2,300**	(2010)
Lifetime risk of maternal death (1 in :)	**300**	(2010)
Women with low BMI (<18.5 kg/m², %)	**–**	**–**
Anaemia, non-pregnant women (<120g/l, %)	**–**	**–**
Antenatal care (at least one visit, %)	**91**	(2008)
Antenatal care (at least four visits, %)	**78**	(2008)
Skilled attendant at birth (%)	**62**	(2008)
Low birthweight (<2,500 grams, %)	**21**	(2008)
Women 20–24 years old who gave birth before age 18 (%)	**7**	(2008)

WATER AND SANITATION

Improved drinking water coverage
Percentage of population, by type of drinking water source, 1990–2010

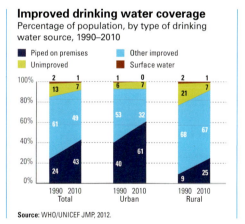

Legend: Piped on premises, Other improved, Unimproved, Surface water

	1990 Total	2010 Total	1990 Urban	2010 Urban	1990 Rural	2010 Rural
	2 / 13 / 61 / 24	1 / 7 / 49 / 43	1 / 6 / 53 / 40	0 / 7 / 32 / 61	2 / 21 / 68 / 9	1 / 7 / 67 / 25

Source: WHO/UNICEF JMP, 2012.

Improved sanitation coverage
Percentage of population, by type of sanitation facility, 1990–2010

Legend: Improved facilities, Shared facilities, Unimproved facilities, Open defecation

	1990 Total	2010 Total	1990 Urban	2010 Urban	1990 Rural	2010 Rural
	16 / 15 / 12 / 57	8 / 2 / 16 / 74	8 / 15 / 69	3 / 17 / 79	23 / 22 / 10 / 45	12 / 3 / 16 / 69

Source: WHO/UNICEF JMP, 2012.

DISPARITIES IN NUTRITION

Indicator	Gender			Residence			Wealth quintile							Source
	Male	Female	Ratio of male to female	Urban	Rural	Ratio of urban to rural	Poorest	Second	Middle	Fourth	Richest	Ratio of richest to poorest	Equity chart	
Stunting prevalence (%)	–	–	–	–	–	–	–	–	–	–	–	–		–
Underweight prevalence (%)	–	–	–	–	–	–	–	–	–	–	–	–		–
Wasting prevalence (%)	–	–	–	–	–	–	–	–	–	–	–	–		–
Women with low BMI (<18.5 kg/m², %)	–	–	–	–	–	–	–	–	–	–	–	–		–
Women with high BMI (≥25 kg/m², %)	–	–	–	–	–	–	–	–	–	–	–	–		–

RWANDA

Total population (000)	**10,943**	(2011)
Total under-five population (000)	**1,912**	(2011)
Total number of births (000)	**449**	(2011)
Under-five mortality rate (per 1,000 live births)	**54**	(2011)
Total number of under-five deaths (000)	**23**	(2011)
Infant mortality rate (per 1,000 live births)	**38**	(2011)
Neonatal mortality rate (per 1,000 live births)	**21**	(2011)
HIV prevalence rate (15–49 years old, %)	**2.9**	(2011)
Population below international poverty line of US$1.25 per day (%)	**63**	(2011)
GNI per capita (US$)	**570**	(2011)
Primary school net attendance ratio (% female, % male)	**89, 86**	(2010)

Causes of under-five deaths, 2010

Globally, undernutrition contributes to more than one third of child deaths

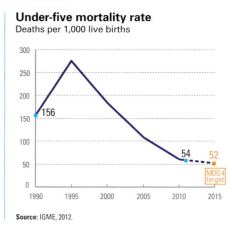

- Others 25%
- Neonatal 34%
- Measles 0%
- Meningitis 2%
- HIV/AIDS 2%
- Injuries 6%
- Malaria 2%
- Pneumonia 17%
- Diarrhoea 12%

Source: WHO/CHERG, 2012.

Under-five mortality rate

Deaths per 1,000 live births

156 ... 54 ... 52 MDG 4 target

Source: IGME, 2012.

Burden of malnutrition (2011)

Stunting country rank	**29**	Stunted (under-fives, 000)	**845**	MDG 1 progress	**On track**
Share of world stunting burden (%)	**<1%**	Wasted (under-fives, 000)	**54**	Underweight (under-fives, 000)	**218**
		Severely wasted (under-fives, 000)	**15**	Overweight (under-fives, 000)	**128**

Stunting trends

Percentage of children <5 years old stunted

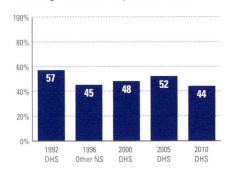

1992 DHS	1996 Other NS	2000 DHS	2005 DHS	2010 DHS
57	45	48	52	44

Stunting disparities

Percentage of children <5 years old stunted, by selected background characteristics

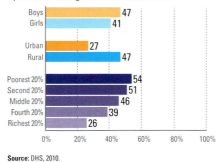

- Boys 47
- Girls 41
- Urban 27
- Rural 47
- Poorest 20% 54
- Second 20% 51
- Middle 20% 46
- Fourth 20% 39
- Richest 20% 26

Source: DHS, 2010.

Underweight trends

Percentage of children <5 years old underweight

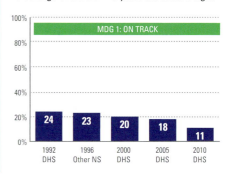

MDG 1: ON TRACK

1992 DHS	1996 Other NS	2000 DHS	2005 DHS	2010 DHS
24	23	20	18	11

Exclusive breastfeeding trends

Percentage of infants <6 months old exclusively breastfed

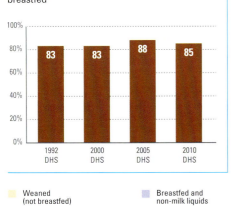

1992 DHS	2000 DHS	2005 DHS	2010 DHS
83	83	88	85

Infant feeding practices, by age

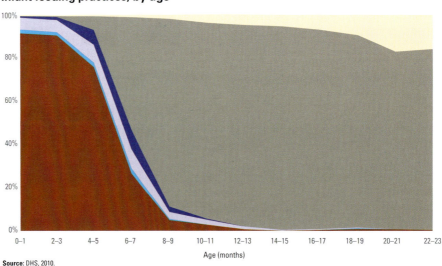

- Weaned (not breastfed)
- Breastfed and solid/semi-solid foods
- Breastfed and other milk/formula
- Breastfed and non-milk liquids
- Breastfed and plain water only
- Exclusively breastfed

Source: DHS, 2010.

Age (months)

RWANDA

ESSENTIAL NUTRITION PRACTICES AND INTERVENTIONS DURING THE LIFE CYCLE

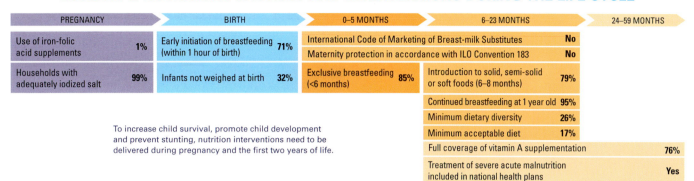

PREGNANCY	BIRTH	0–5 MONTHS	6–23 MONTHS	24–59 MONTHS

Use of iron-folic acid supplements	1%
Households with adequately iodized salt	99%

Early initiation of breastfeeding (within 1 hour of birth)	71%
Infants not weighed at birth	32%

International Code of Marketing of Breast-milk Substitutes	No
Maternity protection in accordance with ILO Convention 183	No
Exclusive breastfeeding (<6 months)	85%

Introduction to solid, semi-solid or soft foods (6–8 months)	79%
Continued breastfeeding at 1 year old	95%
Minimum dietary diversity	26%
Minimum acceptable diet	17%
Full coverage of vitamin A supplementation	76%
Treatment of severe acute malnutrition included in national health plans	Yes

To increase child survival, promote child development and prevent stunting, nutrition interventions need to be delivered during pregnancy and the first two years of life.

MICRONUTRIENTS

Anaemia
Prevalence of anaemia among selected populations

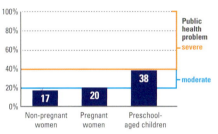

Source: DHS, 2010.

Iodized salt trends*
Percentage of households with adequately iodized salt

3,000 newborns are unprotected against iodine deficiency disorders (2011)

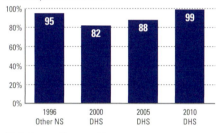

* Estimates may not be comparable.

Vitamin A supplementation
Percentage of children 6–59 months old receiving two doses of vitamin A during calendar year (full coverage)

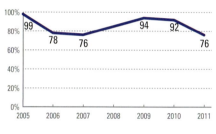

Source: UNICEF, 2012.

MATERNAL NUTRITION AND HEALTH

Maternal mortality ratio, adjusted (per 100,000 live births)	340	(2010)
Maternal mortality ratio, reported (per 100,000 live births)	480	(2010)
Total number of maternal deaths	1,500	(2010)
Lifetime risk of maternal death (1 in :)	54	(2010)
Women with low BMI (<18.5 kg/m², %)	7	(2010)
Anaemia, non-pregnant women (<120g/l, %)	17	(2010)
Antenatal care (at least one visit, %)	98	(2010)
Antenatal care (at least four visits, %)	35	(2010)
Skilled attendant at birth (%)	69	(2010)
Low birthweight (<2,500 grams, %)	7	(2010)
Women 20–24 years old who gave birth before age 18 (%)	5	(2010)

WATER AND SANITATION

Improved drinking water coverage
Percentage of population, by type of drinking water source, 1990–2010

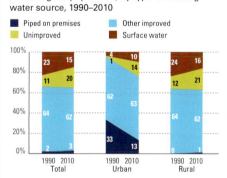

Source: WHO/UNICEF JMP, 2012.

Improved sanitation coverage
Percentage of population, by type of sanitation facility, 1990–2010

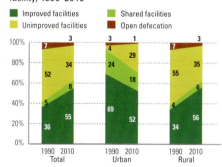

Source: WHO/UNICEF JMP, 2012.

DISPARITIES IN NUTRITION

Indicator	Gender			Residence			Wealth quintile						Equity chart	Source
	Male	Female	Ratio of male to female	Urban	Rural	Ratio of urban to rural	Poorest	Second	Middle	Fourth	Richest	Ratio of richest to poorest		
Stunting prevalence (%)	47	41	1.2	27	47	0.6	54	51	46	39	26	0.5	▪▪▪▪▫	DHS, 2010
Underweight prevalence (%)	13	10	1.3	6	12	0.5	16	14	11	9	5	0.3	▪▪▫▫▫	DHS, 2010
Wasting prevalence (%)	3	2	1.4	4	3	1.3	4	3	2	2	3	0.8	▫▫▫▫▫	DHS, 2010
Women with low BMI (<18.5 kg/m², %)	–	7	–	7	7	0.9	10	9	7	7	5	0.5	▫▫▫▫▫	DHS, 2010
Women with high BMI (≥25 kg/m², %)	–	16	–	25	15	1.7	11	10	14	18	28	2.6	▫▫▫▫▪	DHS, 2010

SIERRA LEONE

DEMOGRAPHICS AND BACKGROUND INFORMATION

Total population (000)	**5,997**	(2011)
Total under-five population (000)	**985**	(2011)
Total number of births (000)	**227**	(2011)
Under-five mortality rate (per 1,000 live births)	**185**	(2011)
Total number of under-five deaths (000)	**42**	(2011)
Infant mortality rate (per 1,000 live births)	**119**	(2011)
Neonatal mortality rate (per 1,000 live births)	**49**	(2011)
HIV prevalence rate (15–49 years old, %)	**1.6**	(2011)
Population below international poverty line of US$1.25 per day (%)	**53**	(2003)
GNI per capita (US$)	**340**	(2011)
Primary school net attendance ratio (% female, % male)	**76, 73**	(2010)

Causes of under-five deaths, 2010
Globally, undernutrition contributes to more than one third of child deaths

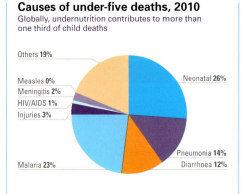

Others 19%
Measles 0%
Meningitis 2%
HIV/AIDS 1%
Injuries 3%
Malaria 23%
Neonatal 26%
Pneumonia 14%
Diarrhoea 12%

Source: WHO/CHERG, 2012.

Under-five mortality rate
Deaths per 1,000 live births

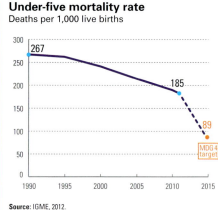

Source: IGME, 2012.

NUTRITIONAL STATUS

Burden of malnutrition (2011)

Stunting country rank	**45**
Share of world stunting burden (%)	**<1%**

Stunted (under-fives, 000)	**438**
Wasted (under-fives, 000)	**84**
Severely wasted (under-fives, 000)	**32**

MDG 1 progress	**No progress**
Underweight (under-fives, 000)	**214**
Overweight (under-fives, 000)	**100**

Stunting trends
Percentage of children <5 years old stunted

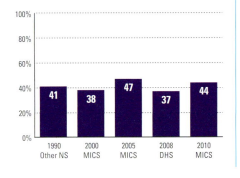

1990 Other NS	2000 MICS	2005 MICS	2008 DHS	2010 MICS
41	38	47	37	44

Stunting disparities
Percentage of children <5 years old stunted, by selected background characteristics

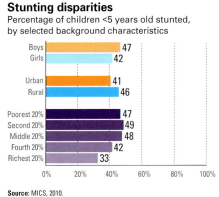

Boys 47
Girls 42
Urban 41
Rural 46
Poorest 20% 47
Second 20% 49
Middle 20% 48
Fourth 20% 42
Richest 20% 33

Source: MICS, 2010.

Underweight trends
Percentage of children <5 years old underweight

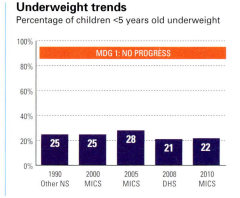

MDG 1: NO PROGRESS

1990 Other NS	2000 MICS	2005 MICS	2008 DHS	2010 MICS
25	25	28	21	22

INFANT AND YOUNG CHILD FEEDING

Exclusive breastfeeding trends
Percentage of infants <6 months old exclusively breastfed

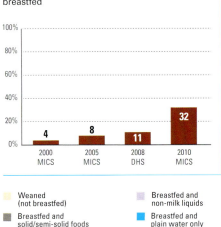

2000 MICS	2005 MICS	2008 DHS	2010 MICS
4	8	11	32

Weaned (not breastfed)
Breastfed and solid/semi-solid foods
Breastfed and other milk/formula
Breastfed and non-milk liquids
Breastfed and plain water only
Exclusively breastfed

Infant feeding practices, by age

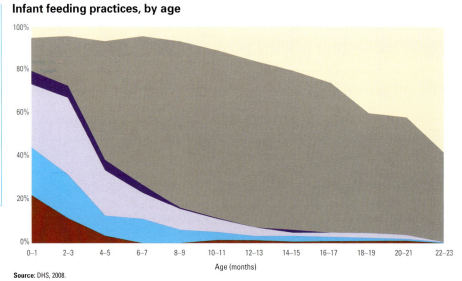

Age (months)

Source: DHS, 2008.

ESSENTIAL NUTRITION PRACTICES AND INTERVENTIONS DURING THE LIFE CYCLE

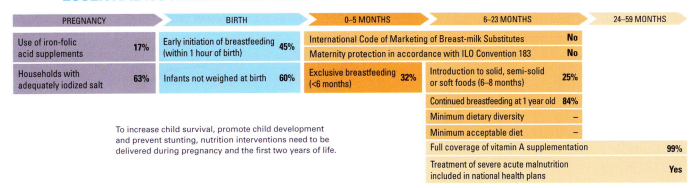

PREGNANCY	BIRTH	0–5 MONTHS	6–23 MONTHS	24–59 MONTHS

| Use of iron-folic acid supplements | 17% |
| Households with adequately iodized salt | 63% |

| Early initiation of breastfeeding (within 1 hour of birth) | 45% |
| Infants not weighed at birth | 60% |

International Code of Marketing of Breast-milk Substitutes	No
Maternity protection in accordance with ILO Convention 183	No
Exclusive breastfeeding (<6 months)	32%

Introduction to solid, semi-solid or soft foods (6–8 months)	25%
Continued breastfeeding at 1 year old	84%
Minimum dietary diversity	–
Minimum acceptable diet	–
Full coverage of vitamin A supplementation	99%
Treatment of severe acute malnutrition included in national health plans	Yes

To increase child survival, promote child development and prevent stunting, nutrition interventions need to be delivered during pregnancy and the first two years of life.

MICRONUTRIENTS

Anaemia
Prevalence of anaemia among selected populations

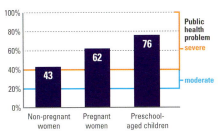

Source: DHS, 2008.

Iodized salt trends*
Percentage of households with adequately iodized salt
85,000 newborns are unprotected against iodine deficiency disorders (2011)

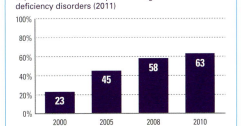

* Estimates may not be comparable.

Vitamin A supplementation
Percentage of children 6–59 months old receiving two doses of vitamin A during calendar year (full coverage)

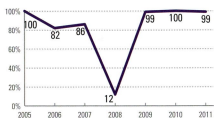

Source: UNICEF, 2012.

MATERNAL NUTRITION AND HEALTH

Maternal mortality ratio, adjusted (per 100,000 live births)	890	(2010)
Maternal mortality ratio, reported (per 100,000 live births)	860	(2008)
Total number of maternal deaths	2,000	(2010)
Lifetime risk of maternal death (1 in :)	23	(2010)
Women with low BMI (<18.5 kg/m², %)	11	(2008)
Anaemia, non-pregnant women (<120g/l, %)	43	(2008)
Antenatal care (at least one visit, %)	93	(2010)
Antenatal care (at least four visits, %)	75	(2010)
Skilled attendant at birth (%)	63	(2010)
Low birthweight (<2,500 grams, %)	11	(2010)
Women 20–24 years old who gave birth before age 18 (%)	38	(2010)

WATER AND SANITATION

Improved drinking water coverage
Percentage of population, by type of drinking water source, 1990–2010

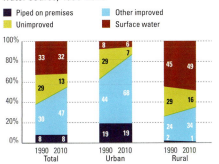

Source: WHO/UNICEF JMP, 2012.

Improved sanitation coverage
Percentage of population, by type of sanitation facility, 1990–2010

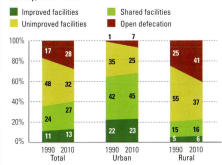

Source: WHO/UNICEF JMP, 2012.

DISPARITIES IN NUTRITION

Indicator	Gender			Residence			Wealth quintile							Source
	Male	Female	Ratio of male to female	Urban	Rural	Ratio of urban to rural	Poorest	Second	Middle	Fourth	Richest	Ratio of richest to poorest	Equity chart	
Stunting prevalence (%)	47	42	1.1	41	46	0.9	47	49	48	42	33	0.7	▪▪▪▪▫	MICS, 2010
Underweight prevalence (%)	24	20	1.2	20	22	0.9	22	25	24	20	15	0.7	▪▫▫▫▫	MICS, 2010
Wasting prevalence (%)	10	7	1.3	10	8	1.2	8	8	9	8	9	1.1	▫▫▫▫▫	MICS, 2010
Women with low BMI (<18.5 kg/m², %)	–	11	–	8	13	0.6	14	14	11	9	9	0.6	▫▫▫▫▫	DHS, 2008
Women with high BMI (≥25 kg/m², %)	–	30	–	42	23	1.8	26	20	26	32	42	1.6	▪▪▫▫▪	DHS, 2008

UNITED REPUBLIC OF TANZANIA

DEMOGRAPHICS AND BACKGROUND INFORMATION

Total population (000)	**46,218**	(2011)
Total under-five population (000)	**8,273**	(2011)
Total number of births (000)	**1,913**	(2011)
Under-five mortality rate (per 1,000 live births)	**68**	(2011)
Total number of under-five deaths (000)	**122**	(2011)
Infant mortality rate (per 1,000 live births)	**45**	(2011)
Neonatal mortality rate (per 1,000 live births)	**25**	(2011)
HIV prevalence rate (15–49 years old, %)	**5.8**	(2011)
Population below international poverty line of US$1.25 per day (%)	**68**	(2007)
GNI per capita (US$)	**540**	(2011)
Primary school net attendance ratio (% female, % male)	**82, 79**	(2010)

Causes of under-five deaths, 2010
Globally, undernutrition contributes to more than one third of child deaths

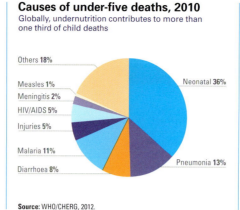

- Others 18%
- Measles 1%
- Meningitis 2%
- HIV/AIDS 5%
- Injuries 5%
- Malaria 11%
- Diarrhoea 8%
- Neonatal 36%
- Pneumonia 13%

Source: WHO/CHERG, 2012.

Under-five mortality rate
Deaths per 1,000 live births

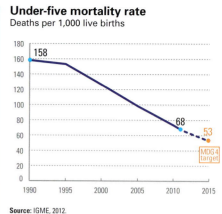

Source: IGME, 2012.

NUTRITIONAL STATUS

Burden of malnutrition (2011)

Stunting country rank	**10**
Share of world stunting burden (%)	**2**

Stunted (under-fives, 000)	**3,475**
Wasted (under-fives, 000)	**397**
Severely wasted (under-fives, 000)	**99**

MDG 1 progress	**On track**
Underweight (under-fives, 000)	**1,307**
Overweight (under-fives, 000)	**455**

Stunting trends
Percentage of children <5 years old stunted

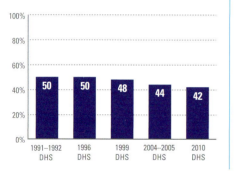

Stunting disparities
Percentage of children <5 years old stunted, by selected background characteristics

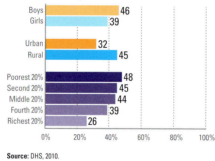

- Boys 46
- Girls 39
- Urban 32
- Rural 45
- Poorest 20% 48
- Second 20% 45
- Middle 20% 44
- Fourth 20% 39
- Richest 20% 26

Source: DHS, 2010.

Underweight trends
Percentage of children <5 years old underweight

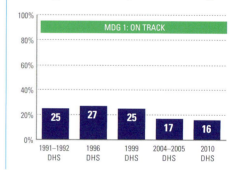

INFANT AND YOUNG CHILD FEEDING

Exclusive breastfeeding trends
Percentage of infants <6 months old exclusively breastfed

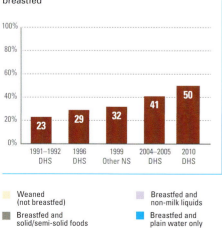

Legend:
- Weaned (not breastfed)
- Breastfed and solid/semi-solid foods
- Breastfed and other milk/formula
- Breastfed and non-milk liquids
- Breastfed and plain water only
- Exclusively breastfed

Infant feeding practices, by age

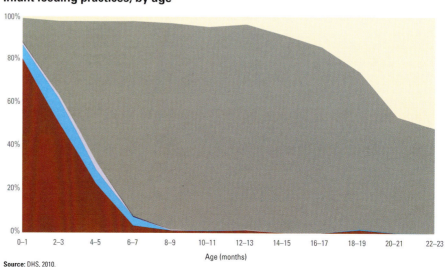

Source: DHS, 2010.

UNITED REPUBLIC OF TANZANIA

ESSENTIAL NUTRITION PRACTICES AND INTERVENTIONS DURING THE LIFE CYCLE

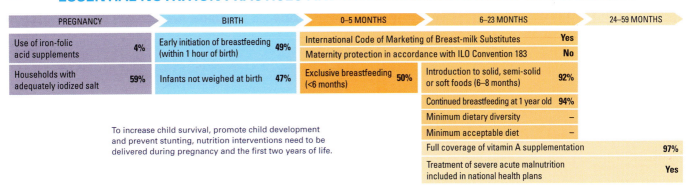

PREGNANCY	BIRTH	0–5 MONTHS	6–23 MONTHS	24–59 MONTHS

Use of iron-folic acid supplements	4%	Early initiation of breastfeeding (within 1 hour of birth)	49%
Households with adequately iodized salt	59%	Infants not weighed at birth	47%

International Code of Marketing of Breast-milk Substitutes	Yes
Maternity protection in accordance with ILO Convention 183	No

Exclusive breastfeeding (<6 months)	50%

To increase child survival, promote child development and prevent stunting, nutrition interventions need to be delivered during pregnancy and the first two years of life.

Introduction to solid, semi-solid or soft foods (6–8 months)	92%
Continued breastfeeding at 1 year old	94%
Minimum dietary diversity	–
Minimum acceptable diet	–
Full coverage of vitamin A supplementation	97%
Treatment of severe acute malnutrition included in national health plans	Yes

MICRONUTRIENTS

Anaemia
Prevalence of anaemia among selected populations

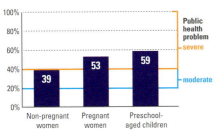

Non-pregnant women: 39
Pregnant women: 53
Preschool-aged children: 59

Public health problem: severe, moderate

Source: DHS, 2010.

Iodized salt trends*
Percentage of households with adequately iodized salt

794,000 newborns are unprotected against iodine deficiency disorders (2011)

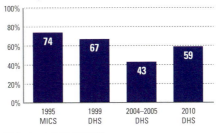

1995 MICS: 74
1999 DHS: 67
2004–2005 DHS: 43
2010 DHS: 59

* Estimates may not be comparable.

Vitamin A supplementation
Percentage of children 6–59 months old receiving two doses of vitamin A during calendar year (full coverage)

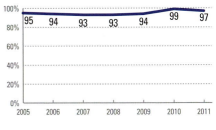

2005: 95
2006: 94
2007: 93
2008: 93
2009: 94
2010: 99
2011: 97

Source: UNICEF, 2012.

MATERNAL NUTRITION AND HEALTH

Maternal mortality ratio, adjusted (per 100,000 live births)	460	(2010)
Maternal mortality ratio, reported (per 100,000 live births)	450	(2010)
Total number of maternal deaths	8,500	(2010)
Lifetime risk of maternal death (1 in :)	38	(2010)
Women with low BMI (<18.5 kg/m², %)	11	(2010)
Anaemia, non-pregnant women (<120g/l, %)	39	(2010)
Antenatal care (at least one visit, %)	88	(2010)
Antenatal care (at least four visits, %)	43	(2010)
Skilled attendant at birth (%)	49	(2010)
Low birthweight (<2,500 grams, %)	8	(2010)
Women 20–24 years old who gave birth before age 18 (%)	28	(2010)

WATER AND SANITATION

Improved drinking water coverage
Percentage of population, by type of drinking water source, 1990–2010

Piped on premises | Other improved
Unimproved | Surface water

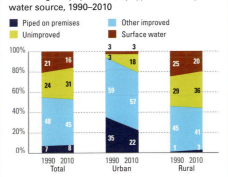

Source: WHO/UNICEF JMP, 2012.

Improved sanitation coverage
Percentage of population, by type of sanitation facility, 1990–2010

Improved facilities | Shared facilities
Unimproved facilities | Open defecation

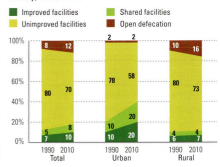

Source: WHO/UNICEF JMP, 2012.

DISPARITIES IN NUTRITION

Indicator	Gender			Residence			Wealth quintile						Equity chart	Source
	Male	Female	Ratio of male to female	Urban	Rural	Ratio of urban to rural	Poorest	Second	Middle	Fourth	Richest	Ratio of richest to poorest		
Stunting prevalence (%)	46	39	1.2	32	45	0.7	48	45	44	39	26	0.5	▪▪▪▪▪	DHS, 2010
Underweight prevalence (%)	17	14	1.2	11	17	0.7	22	18	14	13	9	0.4	▪▪▪▪▪	DHS, 2010
Wasting prevalence (%)	6	4	1.4	5	5	1.0	7	4	4	4	5	0.7	▪▪▪▪▪	DHS, 2010
Women with low BMI (<18.5 kg/m², %)	–	11	–	8	13	0.6	18	13	13	9	7	0.4	▪▪▪▪▪	DHS, 2010
Women with high BMI (≥25 kg/m², %)	–	22	–	36	15	2.4	8	11	14	25	41	5.0	▪▪▪▪▪	DHS, 2010

TIMOR-LESTE

DEMOGRAPHICS AND BACKGROUND INFORMATION

Total population (000)	**1,154**	(2011)
Total under-five population (000)	**202**	(2011)
Total number of births (000)	**44**	(2011)
Under-five mortality rate (per 1,000 live births)	**54**	(2011)
Total number of under-five deaths (000)	**2**	(2011)
Infant mortality rate (per 1,000 live births)	**46**	(2011)
Neonatal mortality rate (per 1,000 live births)	**24**	(2011)
HIV prevalence rate (15–49 years old, %)	**–**	**–**
Population below international poverty line of US$1.25 per day (%)	**37**	(2007)
GNI per capita (US$)	**2,730**	(2010)
Primary school net attendance ratio (% female, % male)	**73, 71**	(2009)

Causes of under-five deaths, 2010
Globally, undernutrition contributes to more than one third of child deaths

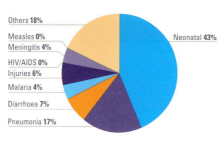

Neonatal **43%**
Others **18%**
Measles **0%**
Meningitis **4%**
HIV/AIDS **0%**
Injuries **6%**
Malaria **4%**
Diarrhoea **7%**
Pneumonia **17%**

Source: WHO/CHERG, 2012.

Under-five mortality rate
Deaths per 1,000 live births

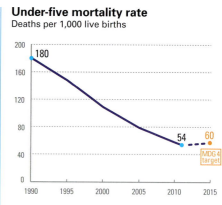

Source: IGME, 2012.

NUTRITIONAL STATUS

Burden of malnutrition (2011)

Stunting country rank	**54**
Share of world stunting burden (%)	**<1%**

Stunted (under-fives, 000)	**118**
Wasted (under-fives, 000)	**38**
Severely wasted (under-fives, 000)	**14**

MDG 1 progress	**No progress**
Underweight (under-fives, 000)	**90**
Overweight (under-fives, 000)	**12**

Stunting trends
Percentage of children <5 years old stunted

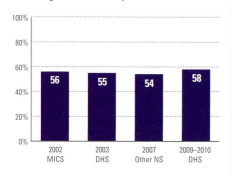

Stunting disparities
Percentage of children <5 years old stunted, by selected background characteristics

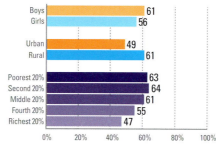

Boys 61
Girls 56
Urban 49
Rural 61
Poorest 20% 63
Second 20% 64
Middle 20% 61
Fourth 20% 55
Richest 20% 47

Source: DHS, 2009–2010.

Underweight trends
Percentage of children <5 years old underweight

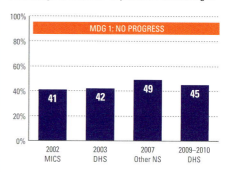

INFANT AND YOUNG CHILD FEEDING

Exclusive breastfeeding trends
Percentage of infants <6 months old exclusively breastfed

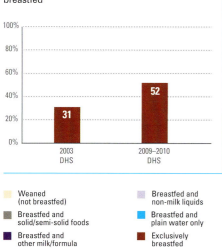

Weaned (not breastfed)
Breastfed and solid/semi-solid foods
Breastfed and other milk/formula
Breastfed and non-milk liquids
Breastfed and plain water only
Exclusively breastfed

Infant feeding practices, by age

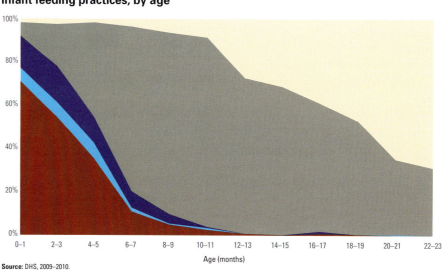

Age (months)

Source: DHS, 2009–2010.

ESSENTIAL NUTRITION PRACTICES AND INTERVENTIONS DURING THE LIFE CYCLE

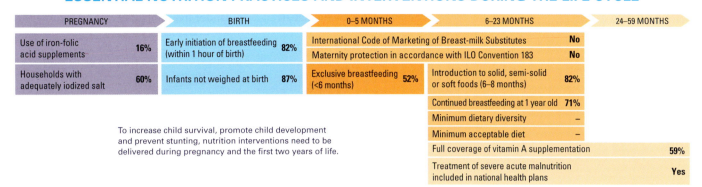

PREGNANCY	BIRTH	0–5 MONTHS	6–23 MONTHS	24–59 MONTHS

Use of iron-folic acid supplements	16%	Early initiation of breastfeeding (within 1 hour of birth)	82%
Households with adequately iodized salt	60%	Infants not weighed at birth	87%

International Code of Marketing of Breast-milk Substitutes	No
Maternity protection in accordance with ILO Convention 183	No
Exclusive breastfeeding (<6 months)	52%

Introduction to solid, semi-solid or soft foods (6–8 months)	82%
Continued breastfeeding at 1 year old	71%
Minimum dietary diversity	–
Minimum acceptable diet	–
Full coverage of vitamin A supplementation	59%
Treatment of severe acute malnutrition included in national health plans	Yes

To increase child survival, promote child development and prevent stunting, nutrition interventions need to be delivered during pregnancy and the first two years of life.

MICRONUTRIENTS

Anaemia
Prevalence of anaemia among selected populations

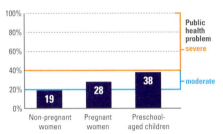

Source: DHS, 2009–2010.

Iodized salt trends*
Percentage of households with adequately iodized salt
18,000 newborns are unprotected against iodine deficiency disorders (2011)

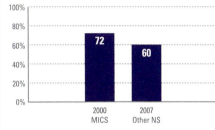

* Estimates may not be comparable.

Vitamin A supplementation
Percentage of children 6–59 months old receiving two doses of vitamin A during calendar year (full coverage)

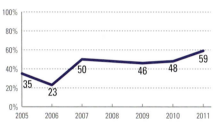

Source: UNICEF, 2012.

MATERNAL NUTRITION AND HEALTH

Maternal mortality ratio, adjusted (per 100,000 live births)	300	(2010)
Maternal mortality ratio, reported (per 100,000 live births)	560	(2009)
Total number of maternal deaths	130	(2010)
Lifetime risk of maternal death (1 in :)	55	(2010)
Women with low BMI (<18.5 kg/m², %)	27	(2009–2010)
Anaemia, non-pregnant women (<120g/l, %)	19	(2009–2010)
Antenatal care (at least one visit, %)	84	(2009–2010)
Antenatal care (at least four visits, %)	55	(2009–2010)
Skilled attendant at birth (%)	29	(2009–2010)
Low birthweight (<2,500 grams, %)	12	(2003)
Women 20–24 years old who gave birth before age 18 (%)	9	(2009–2010)

WATER AND SANITATION

Improved drinking water coverage
Percentage of population, by type of drinking water source, 2010*

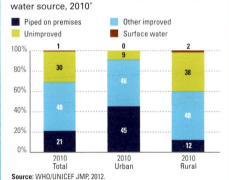

Source: WHO/UNICEF JMP, 2012.
* Insufficient data for generating a trend graph.

Improved sanitation coverage
Percentage of population, by type of sanitation facility, 2010*

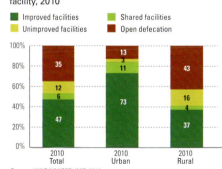

Source: WHO/UNICEF JMP, 2012.
* Insufficient data for generating a trend graph.

DISPARITIES IN NUTRITION

Indicator	Gender			Residence			Wealth quintile							Source
	Male	Female	Ratio of male to female	Urban	Rural	Ratio of urban to rural	Poorest	Second	Middle	Fourth	Richest	Ratio of richest to poorest	Equity chart	
Stunting prevalence (%)	61	56	1.1	49	61	0.8	63	64	61	55	47	0.7	■■■■■	DHS, 2009–2010
Underweight prevalence (%)	46	44	1.0	35	47	0.7	49	48	48	41	35	0.7	▬▬▬▬▬	DHS, 2009–2010
Wasting prevalence (%)	20	17	1.2	15	20	0.8	21	19	20	18	16	0.8	▬▬▬▬▬	DHS, 2009–2010
Women with low BMI (<18.5 kg/m², %)	–	27	–	24	28	0.9	30	29	29	28	22	0.7	■■■■■	DHS, 2009–2010
Women with high BMI (≥25 kg/m², %)	–	5	–	9	4	2.5	2	3	3	6	10	4.5	▬▬▬▬▬	DHS, 2009–2010

ZAMBIA

DEMOGRAPHICS AND BACKGROUND INFORMATION

Total population (000)	13,475	(2011)
Total under-five population (000)	2,510	(2011)
Total number of births (000)	622	(2011)
Under-five mortality rate (per 1,000 live births)	83	(2011)
Total number of under-five deaths (000)	46	(2011)
Infant mortality rate (per 1,000 live births)	53	(2011)
Neonatal mortality rate (per 1,000 live births)	27	(2011)
HIV prevalence rate (15–49 years old, %)	12.5	(2011)
Population below international poverty line of US$1.25 per day (%)	69	(2006)
GNI per capita (US$)	1,160	(2011)
Primary school net attendance ratio (% female, % male)	82, 81	(2007)

Causes of under-five deaths, 2010
Globally, undernutrition contributes to more than one third of child deaths

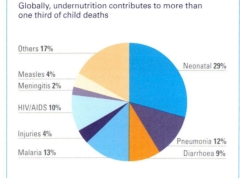

Neonatal 29%
Pneumonia 12%
Diarrhoea 9%
Malaria 13%
Injuries 4%
HIV/AIDS 10%
Meningitis 2%
Measles 4%
Others 17%

Source: WHO/CHERG, 2012.

Under-five mortality rate
Deaths per 1,000 live births

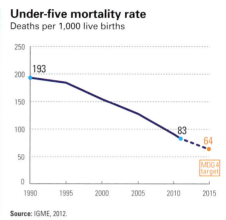

Source: IGME, 2012.

NUTRITIONAL STATUS

Burden of malnutrition (2011)

Stunting country rank	23
Share of world stunting burden (%)	<1%

Stunted (under-fives, 000)	1,140
Wasted (under-fives, 000)	131
Severely wasted (under-fives, 000)	50

MDG 1 progress	**Insufficient progress**
Underweight (under-fives, 000)	366
Overweight (under-fives, 000)	211

Stunting trends
Percentage of children <5 years old stunted

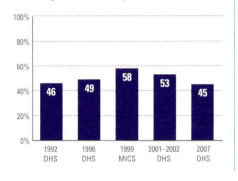

Stunting disparities
Percentage of children <5 years old stunted, by selected background characteristics

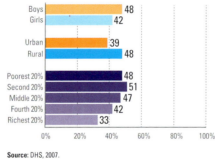

Boys 48
Girls 42
Urban 39
Rural 48
Poorest 20% 48
Second 20% 51
Middle 20% 47
Fourth 20% 42
Richest 20% 33

Source: DHS, 2007.

Underweight trends
Percentage of children <5 years old underweight

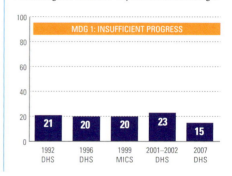

MDG 1: INSUFFICIENT PROGRESS

INFANT AND YOUNG CHILD FEEDING

Exclusive breastfeeding trends
Percentage of infants <6 months old exclusively breastfed

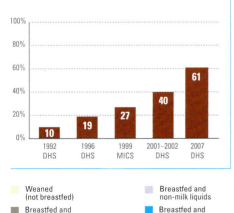

Weaned (not breastfed)

Breastfed and solid/semi-solid foods

Breastfed and other milk/formula

Breastfed and non-milk liquids

Breastfed and plain water only

Exclusively breastfed

Infant feeding practices, by age

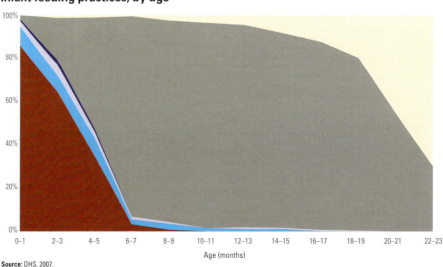

Age (months)

Source: DHS, 2007.

ZAMBIA

ESSENTIAL NUTRITION PRACTICES AND INTERVENTIONS DURING THE LIFE CYCLE

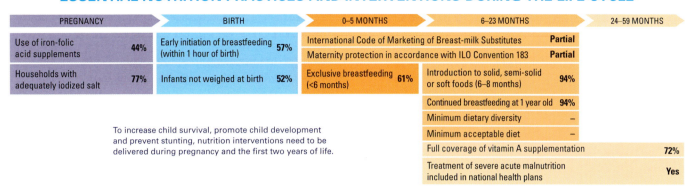

PREGNANCY	BIRTH	0–5 MONTHS	6–23 MONTHS	24–59 MONTHS

Use of iron-folic acid supplements	**44%**	Early initiation of breastfeeding (within 1 hour of birth)	**57%**
Households with adequately iodized salt	**77%**	Infants not weighed at birth	**52%**

International Code of Marketing of Breast-milk Substitutes	**Partial**
Maternity protection in accordance with ILO Convention 183	**Partial**

Exclusive breastfeeding (<6 months)	**61%**	
Introduction to solid, semi-solid or soft foods (6–8 months)		**94%**
Continued breastfeeding at 1 year old		**94%**
Minimum dietary diversity		–
Minimum acceptable diet		–
Full coverage of vitamin A supplementation		**72%**
Treatment of severe acute malnutrition included in national health plans		**Yes**

To increase child survival, promote child development and prevent stunting, nutrition interventions need to be delivered during pregnancy and the first two years of life.

MICRONUTRIENTS

Anaemia
Prevalence of anaemia among selected populations

NO DATA

Iodized salt trends*
Percentage of households with adequately iodized salt
141,000 newborns are unprotected against iodine deficiency disorders (2011)

1995 Other NS	90
1996 DHS	78
2000 MICS	68
2001–2002 DHS	77

* Estimates may not be comparable.

Vitamin A supplementation
Percentage of children 6–59 months old receiving two doses of vitamin A during calendar year (full coverage)

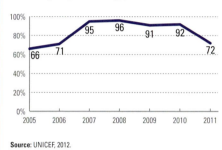

2005	2006	2007	2008	2009	2010	2011
66	71	95	96	91	92	72

Source: UNICEF, 2012.

MATERNAL NUTRITION AND HEALTH

Indicator	Value	Year
Maternal mortality ratio, adjusted (per 100,000 live births)	440	(2010)
Maternal mortality ratio, reported (per 100,000 live births)	590	(2007)
Total number of maternal deaths	2,600	(2010)
Lifetime risk of maternal death (1 in :)	37	(2010)
Women with low BMI (<18.5 kg/m², %)	10	(2007)
Anaemia, non-pregnant women (<120g/l, %)	–	–
Antenatal care (at least one visit, %)	94	(2007)
Antenatal care (at least four visits, %)	60	(2007)
Skilled attendant at birth (%)	47	(2007)
Low birthweight (<2,500 grams, %)	11	(2007)
Women 20–24 years old who gave birth before age 18 (%)	34	(2007)

WATER AND SANITATION

Improved drinking water coverage
Percentage of population, by type of drinking water source, 1990–2010

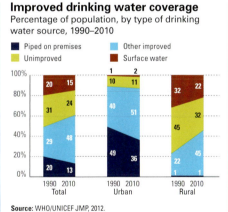

Legend: Piped on premises / Unimproved / Other improved / Surface water

	1990 Total	2010 Total	1990 Urban	2010 Urban	1990 Rural	2010 Rural
Surface water	20	15	10	11	32	22
Other improved	31	24	40	51	45	32
Unimproved	29	48	1	2	22	45
Piped on premises	20	13	49	36	1	1

Source: WHO/UNICEF JMP, 2012.

Improved sanitation coverage
Percentage of population, by type of sanitation facility, 1990–2010

Legend: Improved facilities / Unimproved facilities / Shared facilities / Open defecation

	1990 Total	2010 Total	1990 Urban	2010 Urban	1990 Rural	2010 Rural
Open defecation	25	18	2	2	40	27
Shared facilities	15	20	12	17	16	22
Unimproved facilities	14	14	25	24	7	8
Improved facilities	46	48	61	57	37	43

Source: WHO/UNICEF JMP, 2012.

DISPARITIES IN NUTRITION

Indicator	Gender			Residence			Wealth quintile						Source
	Male	Female	Ratio of male to female	Urban	Rural	Ratio of urban to rural	Poorest	Second	Middle	Fourth	Richest	Ratio of richest to poorest	Equity chart	
Stunting prevalence (%)	48	42	1.1	39	48	0.8	48	51	47	42	33	0.7		DHS, 2007
Underweight prevalence (%)	17	13	1.3	13	15	0.8	16	16	16	13	11	0.7		DHS, 2007
Wasting prevalence (%)	6	5	1.2	4	6	0.8	6	6	5	4	4	0.6		DHS, 2007
Women with low BMI (<18.5 kg/m², %)	–	10	–	8	11	0.7	11	13	12	8	7	0.6		DHS, 2007
Women with high BMI (≥25 kg/m², %)	–	19	–	30	11	2.7	8	9	11	23	35	4.6		DHS, 2007

BOX 6 — Indicators for infant and young child feeding

CORE INDICATORS

- Early initiation of breastfeeding
- Exclusive breastfeeding under 6 months
- Continued breastfeeding at 1 year
- Introduction of solid, semi-solid or soft foods
- Minimum dietary diversity
- Minimum meal frequency
- Minimum acceptable diet*
- Consumption of iron-rich or iron-fortified foods

OPTIONAL INDICATORS

- Children ever breastfed
- Continued breastfeeding at 2 years
- Age-appropriate breastfeeding
- Predominant breastfeeding under 6 months
- Duration of breastfeeding
- Bottle feeding
- Milk feeding frequency of non-breastfed children

*Minimum acceptable diet is a composite indicator of minimum dietary diversity (measures the quality of complementary foods) and minimum meal frequency (a proxy for energy intake). However, several data gaps for minimum dietary diversity and thus minimum acceptable diet exist.

Source: WHO, 2008.

Infant and young child feeding indicators and area graphs

A key step in improving infant and young child nutrition is to effectively measure infant and young child feeding (IYCF) practices. Over the last decade there has been considerable progress in both defining appropriate indicators and improving data collection. In 2002, responding to concerns about the lack of adequate indicators of quality complementary feeding, WHO began a process of reviewing and developing such indicators. At a WHO Global Consensus Meeting in 2007, a revised set of indicators *(Box 6)* were adopted to assess infant and young child feeding practices at the population level and to assist with targeting and support monitoring and evaluation efforts. The country profiles in this report present the latest available data for early initiation of breastfeeding, exclusive breastfeeding under 6 months, continued breastfeeding at 1 year, introduction of solid, semi-solid or soft foods, minimum dietary diversity and minimum acceptable diet.

Interpreting area graphs

The area graphs for infant and young child feeding in the country profiles are based on data collected by Multiple Indicator Cluster Surveys (MICS), Demographic and Health Surveys (DHS) and other national household surveys. These area graphs present the status of infant feeding from birth to 23 months. This information can help identify priorities for improved programming and highlight for policymakers how a country is performing relative to an 'ideal' standard.

In an ideal scenario *(Figure 31)*, almost all children are exclusively breastfed for the recommended first 6 months (burgundy). At 6 months of age, timely introduction of solid, semi-solid and soft foods is recommended. Therefore, there should be a sharp reduction in the number of children who are exclusively breastfed between the 4–5 month and the 6–7 month age groups and an increase in the number of children being breastfed and given solid/semi-solid foods (grey); this grey area should last until children are 22 to 23 months. Feeding children of any age by other means is not desirable (i.e., breastfed and plain water, breastfed and non-milk liquids, breastfed and other milk/formula and not breastfed). Therefore, when these categories are present on a graph they illustrate which inappropriate practices are taking place and they highlight the need for attention to these areas.

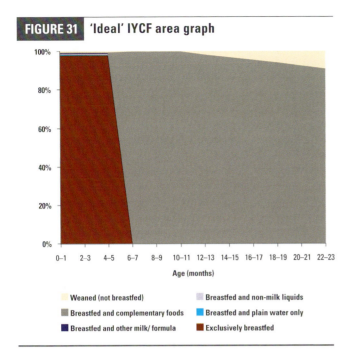

FIGURE 31 'Ideal' IYCF area graph

Age (months)

Weaned (not breastfed) · Breastfed and non-milk liquids
Breastfed and complementary foods · Breastfed and plain water only
Breastfed and other milk/ formula · Exclusively breastfed

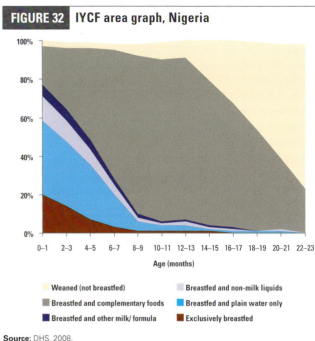

FIGURE 32 IYCF area graph, Nigeria

Age (months)

Weaned (not breastfed) · Breastfed and non-milk liquids
Breastfed and complementary foods · Breastfed and plain water only
Breastfed and other milk/ formula · Exclusively breastfed

Source: DHS, 2008.

A less than optimal scenario can be seen in Figure 32, which shows that while children in Nigeria do receive breastmilk during their first 6 months, only a small proportion of them are exclusively breastfed during this time period. Instead of optimal feeding practices, inappropriate feeding of plain water to children under 6 months of age (light blue area), non-milk liquids (lavender area), other milk/formula (dark blue area) and solid, semi-solid and soft foods (grey area) before 6 months of age continues to occur. Also, after the age of 12 months, there is early cessation of breastfeeding (beige area), which is not recommended. This graph offers clear identification of key areas of less-than-optimal practices that need to be rectified.

Infant feeding practices are closer to recommendations in Rwanda *(Figure 33)*, where rates of exclusive breastfeeding are high in the first 6 months.

Area graphs can be a very useful visual tool for helping national governments and partners assess countrywide infant and young child feeding patterns and clearly see how the practices relate to the 'ideal' standard. The area graphs are most useful for understanding breastfeeding patterns and the timely introduction of complementary foods; they do not reflect the quality of complementary feeding, which is why additional information is required on dietary diversity and frequency. By using area graphs, actions can be prioritized and advocacy and education efforts can be better supported to achieve the best possible infant and young child feeding practices.

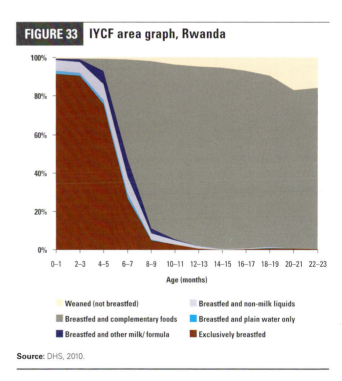

FIGURE 33 IYCF area graph, Rwanda

Age (months)

Weaned (not breastfed) · Breastfed and non-milk liquids
Breastfed and complementary foods · Breastfed and plain water only
Breastfed and other milk/ formula · Exclusively breastfed

Source: DHS, 2010.

All available country area graphs can be found at:<www.childinfo.org/breastfeeding_infantfeeding.html>.

Further information on interpreting infant and young child feeding area graphs can be found at: <www.unicef.org/nutrition/files/Area_graphs_introduction_SinglePg.pdf>.

Definitions of indicators

Indicator		Definition	Numerator	Denominator
Background information				
Child mortality	Under-five mortality rate	Probability of dying between birth and exactly 5 years of age, expressed per 1,000 live births		
	Infant mortality rate	Probability of dying between birth and exactly 1 year of age, expressed per 1,000 live births		
	Neonatal mortality rate	Probability of dying during the first 28 completed days of life, expressed per 1,000 live births		
HIV and AIDS	HIV prevalence (15–49 years)	Percentage of adults (aged 15–49) living with HIV as of 2010		
Poverty	Population below international poverty line of US$ 1.25 per day	Percentage of population living on less than US$ 1.25 per day at 2005 prices, adjusted for purchasing parity		
	Gross national income (GNI) per capita	GNI per capita (formerly GNP per capita) is the gross national income, converted to US dollars using the World Bank Atlas method, divided by the midyear population	Gross national income (GNI)	Midyear population

Indicator		Definition	Numerator	Denominator
Child nutrition				
Anthropometry	Stunting prevalence	Percentage of children 0–59 months who are below minus two (moderate and severe) and below minus three (severe) standard deviations from median height for age of the WHO Child Growth Standards	Number of children 0–59 months who are: (a) below minus two standard deviations (moderate and severe); (b) below minus three standard deviations (severe) from median height for age of the WHO Child Growth Standards	Total number of children 0–59 months
	Underweight prevalence	Percentage of children 0–59 months who are below minus two (moderate and severe) and below minus three (severe) standard deviations from median weight for age of the WHO Child Growth Standards	Number of children 0–59 months who are: (a) below minus two standard deviations (moderate and severe); (b) below minus three standard deviations (severe) from median weight for age of the WHO Child Growth Standards	Total number of children 0–59 months
	Wasting prevalence	Percentage of children 0–59 months who are below minus two (moderate and severe) and below minus three (severe) standard deviations from median weight for height of the WHO Child Growth Standards	Number of children 0–59 months who are: (a) below minus two standard deviations (moderate and severe); (b) below minus three standard deviations (severe) from median weight for height of the WHO Child Growth Standards	Total number of children 0–59 months
	Overweight prevalence	Percentage of children 0–59 months who are above two (moderate and severe) standard deviations from median weight for height of the WHO Child Growth Standards	Number of children 0–59 months who are above two standard deviations (moderate and severe) from median weight for height of the WHO Child Growth Standards	Total number of children 0–59 months

Indicator		Definition	Numerator	Denominator
Infant feeding	Early initiation of breastfeeding (<1 hour of birth)	Percentage of newborns born during the 24 months prior to the survey put to the breast within one hour of birth	Number of women with a live birth during the 24 months prior to the survey who put the newborn to the breast within one hour of birth	Total number of women with a live birth during the same period
	Exclusive breastfeeding rate (<6 months)	Percentage of infants 0–5 months old who were exclusively breastfed	Number of infants 0–5 months old who were exclusively breastfed during the previous day	Total number of infants 0–5 months old
	Introduction to soft, semi-solid and solid foods (6–8 months)	Percentage of infants 6–8 months old who received solid, semi-solid or soft food	Number of infants 6–8 months old who received solid, semi-solid or soft food during the previous day	Total number of infants 6–8 months old
	Continued breastfeeding (12–15 months)	Percentage of children 12–15 months old who are fed breastmilk	Number of children 12–15 months old who were breastfeeding during the previous day	Total number of children 12–15 months old
	Minimum meal frequency	Percentage of children 6–23 months old who received solid, semi-solid or soft foods (including milk feeds for non-breastfed children) the minimum number of times or more [for breastfed children, 'minimum' is defined as two times for infants 6–8 months and three times for children 9–23 months; for non-breastfed children, 'minimum' is defined as four times for children 6–23 months]	Number of breastfed children 6–23 months old, who received solid, semi-solid or soft foods the minimum number of times or more during the previous day	Total number of breastfed children 6–23 months old
			and	
			Number of non-breastfed children 6–23 months old who received solid, semi-solid or soft foods (including milk feeds) the minimum number of times or more during the previous day	Total number of non-breastfed children 6–23 months old
	Minimum dietary diversity	Percentage of children 6–23 months old who receive foods from four or more food groups	Number of children 6–23 months of age who received foods from four or more food groups during the previous day	Total number of children 6–23 months old
	Minimum acceptable diet	Percentage of children 6–23 months old who receive a minimum acceptable diet (apart from breastmilk) (composite indicator)	Number of breastfed children 6–23 months of age who had at least the minimum dietary diversity and the minimum meal frequency during the previous day	Total number of breastfed children 6–23 months old
			and	
			Number of non-breastfed children 6–23 months of age who received at least two milk feedings and had at least the minimum dietary diversity not including milk and the minimum meal frequency during the previous day	Total number of non-breastfed children 6–23 months old
Micronutrients	Vitamin A supplementation (full coverage)	Percentage of children 6–59 months old who received two doses during the calendar year *(refer to 'General note on the data', page 124 for details)*	Number of children 6–59 months old who received two doses of vitamin A during the calendar year	Total number of children 6–59 months old
	Household iodized salt	Percentage of households consuming adequately iodized salt	Number of households with salt testing 15 parts per million or more of iodide/iodate	Total number of households
	Anaemia among preschool-aged children	Percentage of preschool-aged* children with haemoglobin concentration <110 g/L **Age range may vary by country*	Number of preschool-aged children who had a haemoglobin concentration <110 g/L	Total number of preschool-aged children
	Use of iron-folic acid supplements	Percentage of women* who took iron-folic acid supplements for at least 90 days during their last pregnancy prior to the survey **Age range may vary by country*	Number of women who took iron-folic acid supplements for at least 90 days during their last pregnancy in the X years prior to the survey	Total number of women who gave birth during the same period

Indicator		Definition	Numerator	Denominator
Low birthweight	Low birthweight incidence	Percentage of live births that weighed less than 2,500 grams at birth	Number of last live births in the X years prior to the survey weighing below 2,500 grams at birth	Total number of last live births during the same period
	Children not weighed at birth	Percentage of live births that were not weighed at birth	Number of last live births in the X years prior to the survey who were not weighed at birth	Total number of last live births during the same period

Maternal nutrition and health				
Maternal mortality	Maternal mortality ratio (adjusted), *Inter-agency adjusted estimates*	Number of deaths of women from pregnancy-related causes per 100,000 live births, adjusted for under-reporting and misclassification of maternal deaths		
	Maternal mortality ratio (reported), *National authority estimates*	Number of deaths of women from pregnancy-related causes per 100,000 live births		
	Total number of maternal deaths	Total deaths of women while pregnant or within 42 days of termination of pregnancy, irrespective of the duration and site of the pregnancy, from any cause related to or aggravated by the pregnancy or its management but not from accidental or incidental causes		
	Lifetime risk of maternal death	Lifetime risk of maternal death takes into account both the probability of becoming pregnant and the probability of dying as a result of that pregnancy accumulated across a woman's reproductive years		
Nutrition	Body mass index (BMI), female	Percentage of women 15–49 years old* with a body mass index (BMI) of: a) less than 18.5 kg/m² (low), or b) greater than 25 kg/m² (high) *Age range may vary by country	Number of women* 15–49 years old with a BMI a) <18.5 kg/m²; b) >25 kg/m² * Excludes pregnant women and women who gave birth in the two months prior to the survey	Total number of women 15–49 years old * Excludes pregnant women and women who gave birth in the two months prior to the survey
	Anaemia among non-pregnant women	Percentage of non-pregnant women 15–49 years old* with haemoglobin concentration <120 g/L *Age range and marital status may vary by country	Number of non-pregnant women 15–49 years old who had a haemoglobin concentration <120 g/L	Total number of non-pregnant women 15–49 years old
	Anaemia among pregnant women	Percentage of pregnant women* with haemoglobin concentration <110 g/L *Age range and marital status may vary by country	Number of pregnant women 15–49 years old who had a haemoglobin concentration <110 g/L	Total number of pregnant women 15–49 years old

Indicator		Definition	Numerator	Denominator
Maternal health	Antenatal care (at least one visit)	Percentage of women 15–49 years old attended at least once during pregnancy by skilled health personnel for reasons related to the pregnancy	Number of women attended at least once during pregnancy by skilled health personnel (doctor, nurse, midwife or auxiliary midwife) for reasons related to the pregnancy during the X years prior to the survey	Total number of women who had a live birth occurring in the same period
	Antenatal care (four or more visits)	Percentage of women 15–49 years old attended at least four times during pregnancy by any provider (skilled or unskilled) for reasons related to the pregnancy	Number of women attended at least four times during pregnancy by any provider (skilled or unskilled) for reasons related to the pregnancy during the X years prior to the survey	Total number of women who had a live birth occurring in the same period
	Women (20–24 years old) who gave birth before age 18	Percentage of women 20–24 years old who gave birth before age 18		
Delivery care	Skilled attendant at birth	Percentage of live births attended by skilled health personnel	Number of live births to women 15–49 years old in the X years prior to the survey attended during delivery by skilled health personnel (doctor, nurse, midwife or auxiliary midwife)	Total number of live births to women 15–49 years old during the same period

Education

| Education | Primary school net attendance ratio (female, male) | Number of children attending primary or secondary school who are of official primary school age, expressed as a percentage of the total number of children of official primary school age*

 *All data refer to official International Standard Classifications of Education (ISCED) for the primary and secondary education levels and thus may not correspond to a country-specific school system | Number of children attending primary or secondary school who are of official primary school age | Total number of children who are of official primary school age |

Water and sanitation

Water	Drinking water coverage	Percentage of the population using improved drinking-water sources	*Piped into dwelling, plot or yard –* Number of household members living in households using piped drinking-water connection located inside the user's dwelling, plot or yard	Total number of household members in households surveyed
			Other improved – Number of household members living in households using public taps or standpipes, tube wells or boreholes, protected dug wells, protected springs or rainwater collection	
		Percentage of the population using unimproved drinking-water sources	*Unimproved –* Number of household members living in households using unprotected dug well; unprotected spring cart with small tank/drum; tanker truck; surface water (river dam, lake, pond, stream, canal, irrigation channels); and bottled water	

Indicator		Definition	Numerator	Denominator
Sanitation	Sanitation coverage	Percentage of the population using improved sanitation facilities	*Improved* – Number of household members using improved sanitation facilities (facilities that ensure hygienic separation of human excreta from human contact), including flush or pour flush toilet/latrine to piped sewer system, septic tank or pit latrine; ventilated improved pit latrine; pit latrine with slab; and composting toilet	Total number of household members in households surveyed
		Percentage of the population using unimproved sanitation facilities	*Shared* – Number of household members using sanitation facilities of an otherwise acceptable type shared between two or more households including public toilets	
			Unimproved – Number of household members using sanitation facilities that do not ensure hygienic separation of human excreta from human contact, including pit latrines without a slab or platform, hanging latrines and bucket latrines	
			Open defecation – Number of household members defecating in fields, forests, bushes, bodies of water or other open spaces	

Policies and systems

Policies	International Code of Marketing of Breast-milk Substitutes	National regulations adopted on all provisions of the International Code of Marketing of Breast-milk Substitutes and subsequent World Health Assembly resolutions	*Yes:* All provisions of the International Code adopted in legislation	
			Partial: Voluntary agreements or some provisions of the International Code adopted in legislation	
			No: No legislation and no voluntary agreements adopted in relation to the International Code	
	Treatment of severe acute malnutrition included in national health plans	Indicates the status of each country regarding inclusion of treatment of severe acute malnutrition in national health plans	*Yes:* Treatment of SAM included in national health plans	
			Partial: Treatment of SAM at some stage of inclusion into national health plans (e.g., process started, pending finalization)	
			No: National health plans do not include treatment of SAM, and the process of development has not been initiated	
	Maternity protection in accordance with International Labour Organization (ILO) Convention no. 183	ILO Convention no. 183 ratified by the country	*Yes:* ILO Convention no. 183 ratified	
			Partial: ILO Convention no. 183 not ratified but previous maternity convention (no. 3 or no. 103) ratified	
			No: No ratification of any maternity protection convention	

Data sources

Demographics and background indicators

Total population, total under-five population, total number of births – United Nations, Department of Economic and Social Affairs, Population Division. *World Population Prospects: The 2010 revision*, CD-ROM Edition, <http://esa.un.org/unpd/wpp/index.htm>.

Under-five mortality rate, infant mortality rate, total number of under-five deaths – United Nations Inter-agency Group for Child Mortality Estimation (IGME). UNICEF/WHO/World Bank/United Nations Population Division, 2012.

Causes of under-five deaths – World Health Organization. Child Health Epidemiology Reference Group (CHERG), 2012.

Neonatal mortality rate – World Health Organization. Civil registrations, surveillance systems and household surveys.

HIV prevalence (15–49 years) – Joint United Nations Programme on HIV/AIDS (UNAIDS). *Report on the Global AIDS Epidemic 2012.*

Population below international poverty line of US $1.25 per day, gross national income (GNI) per capita – World Bank.

Primary school net attendance rate (female, male) – United Nations Children's Fund, based on Demographic and Health Surveys, Multiple Indicator Cluster Surveys, other national household surveys.

Child nutrition

Stunting prevalence, underweight prevalence, wasting prevalence, overweight prevalence – United Nations Children's Fund, based on Demographic and Health Surveys, Multiple Indicator Cluster Surveys, other national household surveys.

Early initiation of breastfeeding (<1 hour of birth), exclusive breastfeeding rate (<6 months), introduction to soft, semi-soft and solid foods (6–8 months), continued breastfeeding (12–15 months) – United Nations Children's Fund, based on Demographic and Health Surveys, Multiple Indicator Cluster Surveys, other national household surveys.

Minimum meal frequency, dietary diversity, minimum acceptable diet – United Nations Children's Fund, special data compilation by Nutrition Section, based on Demographic and Health Surveys, Multiple Indicator Cluster Surveys, other national household surveys.

Vitamin A supplementation (full coverage) – United Nations Children's Fund, based on National Immunization Days and routine reporting, Demographic and Health Surveys, Multiple Indicator Cluster Surveys.

Household iodized salt – United Nations Children's Fund, based on Demographic and Health Surveys (DHS), Multiple Indicator Cluster Surveys (MICS), other national household surveys.

Anaemia among preschool-aged children, use of iron-folic acid supplements – United Nations Children's Fund, special data compilation by Nutrition Section, based on DHS, MICS and other national household surveys.

Low birthweight incidence, children not weighed at birth – United Nations Children's Fund, based on Demographic and Health Surveys, Multiple Indicator Cluster Surveys, other national household surveys.

Maternal nutrition and health

Maternal mortality ratio (adjusted), total number of maternal deaths, lifetime risk of maternal death – Maternal Mortality Estimation Inter-agency Group (MMEIG). WHO/UNICEF/United Nations Population Fund/World Bank, 2012.

Maternal mortality ratio (reported) – United Nations Children's Fund, based on vital registration systems, routine reporting, Demographic and Health Surveys, Multiple Indicator Cluster Surveys, and other national household surveys.

Body mass index (BMI), female, anaemia among non-pregnant women, anaemia among pregnant women – United Nations Children's Fund, special data compilation by Nutrition Section, based on Demographic and Health Surveys, Multiple Indicator Cluster Surveys, other national household surveys.

Antenatal care (at least one visit), antenatal care (four or more visits), women 20–24 years old who gave birth before age 18, skilled attendant at birth – United Nations Children's Fund, based on Demographic and Health Surveys, Multiple Indicator Cluster Surveys, other national household surveys.

Water and sanitation

Drinking water coverage, sanitation coverage – World Health Organization/United Nations Children's Fund, Joint Monitoring Programme (JMP) for Water Supply and Sanitation, 2012.

Policies and systems

International Code of Marketing of Breast-milk Substitutes – United Nations Children's Fund, special data compilation by Nutrition Section in October 2012.

Treatment of severe acute malnutrition included in national health plans – United Nations Children's Fund, special data compilation by Nutrition Section for global SAM update in December 2011.

Maternity protection in accordance with International Labour Organization – International Labour Organization. NORMLEX (Information System on International Labour Standards), accessed October 2012.

STATISTICAL TABLES

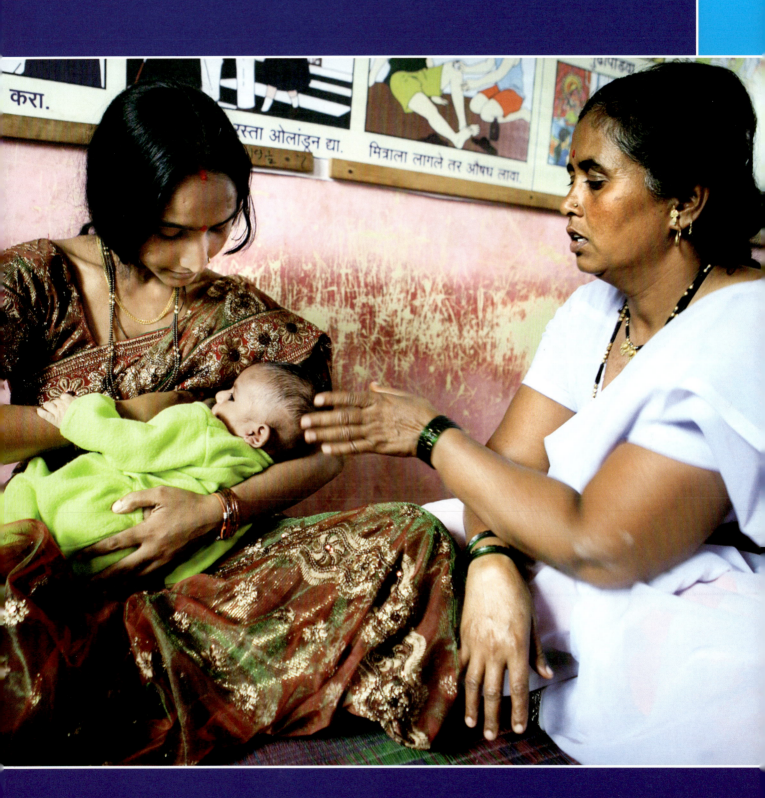

Table 1. Country ranking based on number of stunted children

Ranking[β]	Countries and areas	Stunting prevalence (%) 2007–2011*	Number of stunted children^ (thousands) 2011	Share of world total (%) 2011	Under-five mortality rate 2011
1	India	48 x	61,723	37.9	61
2	Nigeria	41	11,049	6.8	124
3	Pakistan	44	9,663	5.9	72
4	China	10	8,059	5.0	15
5	Indonesia	36	7,547	4.6	32
6	Bangladesh	41	5,958	3.7	46
7	Ethiopia	44	5,291	3.3	77
8	Democratic Republic of the Congo	43	5,228	3.2	168
9	Philippines	32 y	3,602	2.2	25
10	United Republic of Tanzania	42	3,475	2.1	68
11	Egypt	29	2,628	1.6	21
12	Kenya	35	2,403	1.5	73
13	Uganda	33	2,219	1.4	90
14	Sudan[+]	35	1,744	1.1	86
15	Madagascar	50	1,693	1.0	62
16	Mozambique	43	1,651	1.0	103
17	Viet Nam	23	1,635	1.0	22
18	Niger	51 y	1,632	1.0	125
19	Myanmar	35	1,399	<1	62
20	Nepal	41	1,397	<1	48
21	Malawi	47	1,334	<1	83
22	South Africa	24	1,191	<1	47
23	Zambia	45	1,140	<1	83
24	Burkina Faso	35	1,068	<1	146
25	Guatemala	48 y	1,052	<1	30
26	Cameroon	33	1,009	<1	127
27	Ghana	28	1,006	<1	78
28	Angola	29 y	991	<1	158
29	Rwanda	44	845	<1	54
30	Côte d'Ivoire	27 y	818	<1	115
31	Turkey	12	799	<1	15
32	Chad	39	793	<1	169
33	Burundi	58	703	<1	139
34	Guinea	40	678	<1	126
35	Syrian Arab Republic	28	673	<1	15
36	Cambodia	40	601	<1	43
37	Colombia	13	595	<1	18
38	Peru	20	566	<1	18
39	Senegal	27	564	<1	65
40	Democratic People's Republic of Korea	32	553	<1	33
41	Zimbabwe	32	550	<1	67
42	South Sudan[+]	31	463	<1	121
43	Venezuela (Bolivarian Republic of)	16	458	<1	15
44	Morocco	15	455	<1	33
45	Sierra Leone	44	438	<1	185
46	Tajikistan	39	346	<1	63
47	Bolivia (Plurinational State of)	27	333	<1	51
48	Sri Lanka	17	326	<1	12
49	Liberia	42 y	291	<1	78
50	Central African Republic	41	270	<1	164
51	Togo	30	258	<1	110
52	Nicaragua	22	149	<1	26
53	El Salvador	19 y	121	<1	15
54	Timor-Leste	58	118	<1	54
55	Mauritania	23 y	117	<1	112
56	Lesotho	39	108	<1	86
57	Dominican Republic	10	103	<1	25
58	Namibia	29	83	<1	42
59	Guinea-Bissau	32	79	<1	161
60	Botswana	31	72	<1	26
61	Gambia	24	71	<1	101
62	Panama	19 y	66	<1	20
63	Jordan	8	65	<1	21
64	Mongolia	16	51	<1	31

Table 1. Country ranking based on number of stunted children

| Ranking[β] | Countries and areas | Stunting | | | Under-five mortality rate 2011 |
		Stunting prevalence (%) 2007–2011*	Number of stunted children^ (thousands) 2011	Share of world total (%) 2011	
65	Swaziland	31	49	<1	104
66	Armenia	19	43	<1	18
67	Albania	19	39	<1	14
68	Serbia	7	36	<1	7
69	Djibouti	31 y	35	<1	90
70	Georgia	11	29	<1	21
71	Oman	10	28	<1	9
72	Solomon Islands	33	27	<1	22
73	Bhutan	34	23	<1	54
74	Costa Rica	6	20	<1	10
75	Guyana	18	11	<1	36
76	Jamaica	4	9	<1	18
77	Sao Tome and Principe	29	7	<1	89
78	The former Yugoslav Republic of Macedonia	5	5	<1	10
79	Maldives	19	5	<1	11
80	Nauru	24	0	<1	40
81	Tuvalu	10	0	<1	30

DEFINITIONS OF THE INDICATORS

Stunting prevalence – Moderate and severe: Percentage of children aged 0–59 months who are below minus two standard deviations from median height-for-age of the World Health Organization (WHO) Child Growth Standards.

Under-five mortality rate – Probability of dying between birth and exactly 5 years of age, expressed per 1,000 live births.

MAIN DATA SOURCES

Stunting prevalence – Demographic and Health Surveys (DHS), Multiple Indicator Cluster Surveys (MICS), other national household surveys, WHO and UNICEF.

Number of stunted children – Calculated by UNICEF based on stunting prevalence and under-five population from United Nations Population Division.

Under-five mortality rate – United Nations Inter-agency Group for Child Mortality Estimation (IGME). UNICEF/WHO/World Bank/United Nations Population Division, 2012.

NOTES

β   Ranking of 81 countries presented is based on the most recent available survey data (2007–2011).

*   Data refer to the most recent year available during the period specified in the column heading.

x   Data refer to years or periods other than those specified in the column heading.

y   Data differ from the standard definition or refer to only part of a country.

^   Calculated based on prevalence of stunting estimate (moderate and severe) applied to the under-five population estimate.

+   Under-five population estimated by UNICEF.

Table 2. Demographic and nutritional status indicators

Countries and areas	Under-five mortality rate 2011	Under-five population (thousands) 2011	Low birthweight (%) 2007–2011*	% of under-fives (2007–2011*) suffering from: Stunting moderate & severe	Wasting moderate & severe	Underweight moderate & severe	Overweight moderate & severe
Afghanistan	101	5,686	–	59 x	9 x	33 x	5 x
Albania	14	203	7 x	19	9	5	23
Algeria	30	3,464	6 x	15 x	4 x	3 x	13 x
Andorra	3	4	–	–	–	–	–
Angola	158	3,393	12 x	29 y	8 y	16 y	–
Antigua and Barbuda	8	8	5	–	–	–	–
Argentina	14	3,423	7	8 x	1 x	2 x	10 x
Armenia	18	225	7	19	4	5	17
Australia	5	1,504	7 x	–	–	–	–
Austria	4	381	7 x	–	–	–	–
Azerbaijan	45	846	10 x	25 x	7 x	8 x	14 x
Bahamas	16	27	11	–	–	–	–
Bahrain	10	102	–	–	–	–	–
Bangladesh	46	14,421	22 x	41	16	36	2
Barbados	20	15	12	–	–	–	–
Belarus	6	527	4 x	4 x	2 x	1 x	10 x
Belgium	4	619	–	–	–	–	–
Belize	17	37	14	22 x	2 x	4 x	14 x
Benin	106	1,546	15 x	43 x	8 x	18 x	11 x
Bhutan	54	70	10	34	6	13	8
Bolivia (Plurinational State of)	51	1,230	6	27	1	4	9
Bosnia and Herzegovina	8	167	5 x	10 x	4 x	1 x	26 x
Botswana	26	229	13	31	7	11	11
Brazil	16	14,662	8	7 x	2 x	2 x	7
Brunei Darussalam	7	37	–	–	–	–	–
Bulgaria	12	378	9	–	–	–	14 x
Burkina Faso	146	3,047	16 x	35	11	26	–
Burundi	139	1,221	11 x	58	6	29	3
Cambodia	43	1,505	11	40	11	28	2
Cameroon	127	3,102	11 x	33	6	15	6
Canada	6	1,936	6 x	–	–	–	–
Cape Verde	21	50	6 x	–	–	–	–
Central African Republic	164	658	14	41	7	24	2
Chad	169	2,047	20	39	16	30	3
Chile	9	1,222	6	–	–	–	10
China	15	82,205	3	10	3	4	7
Colombia	18	4,509	6 x	13	1	3	5
Comoros	79	124	25 x	–	–	–	22 x
Congo	99	637	13 x	30 x	8 x	11 x	9 x
Cook Islands	10	2	3 x	–	–	–	–
Costa Rica	10	359	7	6	1	1	8
Côte d'Ivoire	115	2,992	17 x	27 y	5 y	16 y	–
Croatia	5	215	5 x	–	–	–	–
Cuba	6	543	5	–	–	–	–
Cyprus	3	65	–	–	–	–	–
Czech Republic	4	567	7 x	–	–	–	4 x
Democratic People's Republic of Korea	33	1,706	6	32	5	19	–
Democratic Republic of the Congo	168	12,037	10	43	9	24	–
Denmark	4	327	5 x	–	–	–	–
Djibouti	90	115	10 x	31 y	10 y	23 y	10 x
Dominica	12	6	10	–	–	–	–
Dominican Republic	25	1,051	11	10	2	3	8
Ecuador	23	1,469	8	–	–	6 x	5 x
Egypt	21	9,092	13	29	7	6	21
El Salvador	15	631	9	19 y	1 y	6 y	6
Equatorial Guinea	118	111	13 x	35 x	3 x	11 x	8 x
Eritrea	68	879	14 x	44 x	15 x	35 x	2 x
Estonia	4	80	4 x	–	–	–	–
Ethiopia	77	11,915	20 x	44	10	29	2
Fiji	16	91	10 x	–	–	–	–
Finland	3	303	4 x	–	–	–	–
France	4	3,985	–	–	–	–	–
Gabon	66	188	14 x	25 x	4 x	8 x	6 x
Gambia	101	292	10	24	10	18	2

Table 2. Demographic and nutritional status indicators ▶

Countries and areas	Under-five mortality rate 2011	Under-five population (thousands) 2011	Low birthweight (%) 2007–2011*	% of under-fives (2007–2011*) suffering from: Stunting[θ] moderate & severe	Wasting[θ] moderate & severe	Underweight[θ] moderate & severe	Overweight[θ] moderate & severe
Georgia	21	258	5	11	2	1	20
Germany	4	3,504	–	–	–	–	4 x
Ghana	78	3,591	13	28	9	14	6
Greece	4	600	–	–	–	–	–
Grenada	13	10	9	–	–	–	–
Guatemala	30	2,192	11	48 y	1 y	13 y	5
Guinea	126	1,691	12 x	40	8	21	–
Guinea-Bissau	161	244	11	32	6	18	3
Guyana	36	60	14	18	5	11	6
Haiti	70	1,245	25 x	29 x	10 x	18 x	4 x
Holy See	–	–	–	–	–	–	–
Honduras	21	975	10 x	29 x	1 x	8 x	6 x
Hungary	6	493	9 x	–	–	–	–
Iceland	3	24	4 x	–	–	–	–
India	61	128,542	28 x	48 x	20 x	43 x	2 x
Indonesia	32	21,210	9	36	13	18	14
Iran (Islamic Republic of)	25	6,269	7 x	–	–	–	–
Iraq	38	5,294	15 x	26 x	6 x	6 x	15 x
Ireland	4	370	–	–	–	–	–
Israel	4	754	8 x	–	–	–	–
Italy	4	2,910	–	–	–	–	–
Jamaica	18	254	12 x	4	2	2	–
Japan	3	5,418	8 x	–	–	–	–
Jordan	21	817	13	8	2	2	7
Kazakhstan	28	1,726	6 x	17 x	5 x	4 x	17 x
Kenya	73	6,805	8	35	7	16	5
Kiribati	47	10	–	–	–	–	–
Kuwait	11	282	–	–	–	–	9
Kyrgyzstan	31	624	5 x	18 x	3 x	2 x	11 x
Lao People's Democratic Republic	42	682	11 x	48 x	7 x	31 x	1 x
Latvia	8	117	5 x	–	–	–	–
Lebanon	9	328	12	–	–	–	17 x
Lesotho	86	276	11	39	4	13	7
Liberia	78	700	14	42 y	3 y	15 y	4
Libya	16	717	–	–	–	–	22
Liechtenstein	–	2	–	–	–	–	–
Lithuania	6	173	4 x	–	–	–	–
Luxembourg	3	29	8 x	–	–	–	–
Madagascar	62	3,378	16	50	15 x	36 x	–
Malawi	83	2,829	13 x	47	4	13	9
Malaysia	7	2,796	11	17 x	–	13 x	–
Maldives	11	26	22 x	19	11	17	7
Mali	176	2,995	19 x	38 x	15 x	27 x	–
Malta	6	20	6 x	–	–	–	–
Marshall Islands	26	5	18	–	–	–	–
Mauritania	112	522	34	23 y	12 y	20 y	–
Mauritius	15	81	14 x	–	–	–	–
Mexico	16	10,943	7	16 x	2 x	3 x	8 x
Micronesia (Federated States of)	42	13	18 x	–	–	–	–
Monaco	4	2	–	–	–	–	–
Mongolia	31	317	5	16	2	5	14 x
Montenegro	7	39	4 x	7 x	4 x	2 x	16 x
Morocco	33	3,048	15 x	15	2	3	11
Mozambique	103	3,877	16	43	6	15	7
Myanmar	62	3,981	9	35	8	23	3
Namibia	42	288	16 x	29	8	17	5
Nauru	40	1	27	24	1	5	3
Nepal	48	3,453	18	41	11	29	1
Netherlands	4	907	–	–	–	–	–
New Zealand	6	320	6 x	–	–	–	–
Nicaragua	26	684	9	22	1	6	6
Niger	125	3,196	27 x	51 y	12 y	39 y	4 x
Nigeria	124	27,195	12	41	14	23	11
Niue	21	0	0 x	–	–	–	–

◀ Table 2. Demographic and nutritional status indicators

Countries and areas	Under-five mortality rate 2011	Under-five population (thousands) 2011	Low birthweight (%) 2007–2011*	% of under-fives (2007–2011*) suffering from:			
				Stunting[θ] moderate & severe	Wasting[θ] moderate & severe	Underweight[θ] moderate & severe	Overweight[θ] moderate & severe
Norway	3	309	5 x	–	–	–	–
Oman	9	290	12	10	7	9	2
Pakistan	72	22,064	32	44	15	32	6
Palau	19	2	–	–	–	–	–
Panama	20	345	10 x	19 y	1 y	4 y	–
Papua New Guinea	58	975	11 x	43 x	5 x	18 x	3 x
Paraguay	22	744	6	18 x	1 x	3 x	7 x
Peru	18	2,902	8	20	0	4	–
Philippines	25	11,161	21	32 y	7 y	22 y	3
Poland	6	2,008	6 x	–	–	–	–
Portugal	3	501	8 x	–	–	–	–
Qatar	8	97	–	–	–	–	–
Republic of Korea	5	2,488	4 x	–	–	–	–
Republic of Moldova	16	223	6 x	10 x	5 x	3 x	9 x
Romania	13	1,093	8 x	13 x	4 x	4 x	8 x
Russian Federation	12	8,264	6	–	–	–	–
Rwanda	54	1,909	7	44	3	11	7
Saint Kitts and Nevis	7	5	8	–	–	–	–
Saint Lucia	16	15	11	–	–	–	–
Saint Vincent and the Grenadines	21	9	8	–	–	–	–
Samoa	19	22	10	–	–	–	–
San Marino	2	2	–	–	–	–	–
Sao Tome and Principe	89	24	8 x	29	11	13	12
Saudi Arabia	9	3,186	–	–	–	–	6 x
Senegal	65	2,125	19	27	10	18	3
Serbia	7	551	5	7	4	2	16
Seychelles	14	14	–	–	–	–	–
Sierra Leone	185	984	11	44	9	22	10
Singapore	3	238	8 x	4 x	4 x	3 x	3 x
Slovakia	8	281	7 x	–	–	–	–
Slovenia	3	102	–	–	–	–	–
Solomon Islands	22	81	13	33	4	12	3
Somalia	180	1,701	–	42 x	13 x	32 x	5 x
South Africa	47	4,989	–	24	5	9	–
South Sudan[δ]	121	–	–	31	23	28	–
Spain	4	2,546	–	–	–	–	–
Sri Lanka	12	1,886	17	17	15	21	1
State of Palestine	22	635	7 x	–	–	–	
Sudan[δ]	86	–	–	35	16	32	–
Suriname	30	47	11 x	11 x	5 x	7 x	4 x
Swaziland	104	158	9	31	1	6	11
Sweden	3	562	–	–	–	–	–
Switzerland	4	382	–	–	–	–	–
Syrian Arab Republic	15	2,446	10	28	12	10	18
Tajikistan	63	883	10 x	39	7	15	–
Thailand	12	4,270	7	16 x	5 x	7 x	8 x
The former Yugoslav Republic of Macedonia	10	112	6	5	2	1	16 x
Timor-Leste	54	201	12 x	58	19	45	6
Togo	110	870	11	30	5	17	2
Tonga	15	14	3 x	–	–	–	–
Trinidad and Tobago	28	96	19 x	–	–	–	5 x
Tunisia	16	885	5 x	9 x	3 x	3 x	9 x
Turkey	15	6,489	11	12	1	2	9 x
Turkmenistan	53	499	4 x	19 x	7 x	8 x	–
Tuvalu	30	1	6	10	3	2	6
Uganda	90	6,638	14 x	33	5	14	3
Ukraine	10	2,465	4	–	–	–	–
United Arab Emirates	7	451	–	–	–	–	–
United Kingdom	5	3,858	8 x	–	–	–	–
United Republic of Tanzania	68	8,267	8	42	5	16	6
United States	8	21,629	8 x	3 x	0 x	1 x	8 x
Uruguay	10	245	9	15 x	2 x	5 x	9 x
Uzbekistan	49	2,802	5 x	19 x	4 x	4 x	13 x
Vanuatu	13	34	10	–	–	–	5

Table 2. Demographic and nutritional status indicators

Countries and areas	Under-five mortality rate	Under-five population (thousands)	Low birthweight (%)	% of under-fives (2007–2011*) suffering from:			
				Stunting[θ]	Wasting[θ]	Underweight[θ]	Overweight[θ]
	2011	2011	2007–2011*	moderate & severe	moderate & severe	moderate & severe	moderate & severe
Venezuela (Bolivarian Republic of)	15	2,935	8	16	5	4	6
Viet Nam	22	7,202	5	23	4	12	–
Yemen	77	4,179	–	58 x	15 x	43 x	5 x
Zambia	83	2,509	11	45	5	15	8
Zimbabwe	67	1,706	11	32	3	10	6
Memorandum							
Sudan and South Sudan[δ]	–	6,472	–	–	–	–	5 x
SUMMARY INDICATORS#							
Sub-Saharan Africa	109	140,617	12	40	9	21	7
Eastern and Southern Africa	84	63,188	–	40	7	18	5
West and Central Africa	132	70,843	12	39	12	23	9
Middle East and North Africa	36	48,169	–	20	9	8	12
South Asia	62	176,150	28	39	16	33	3
East Asia and the Pacific	20	141,248	6	12	4	6	5
Latin America and the Caribbean	19	52,898	8	12	2	3	7
CEE/CIS	21	28,590	7	12	1	2	16
Least developed countries	98	124,162	–	38	10	23	4
World	51	638,681	15	26	8	16	7

\# For a complete list of countries and areas in the regions and subregions, see page 124.

δ Due to the cession in July 2011 of the Republic of South Sudan by the Republic of the Sudan, and its subsequent admission to the United Nations on 14 July 2011, disaggregated data for Sudan and South Sudan as separate States are not yet available for all indicators. In these cases, aggregated data are presented for Sudan pre-cession (see Memorandum item).

DEFINITIONS OF THE INDICATORS

Under-five mortality rate – Probability of dying between birth and exactly 5 years of age, expressed per 1,000 live births.

Low birthweight – Percentage of infants weighing less than 2,500 grams at birth.

Stunting – Moderate and severe: Percentage of children aged 0–59 months who are below minus two standard deviations from median height-for-age of the World Health Organization (WHO) Child Growth Standards.

Wasting – Moderate and severe: Percentage of children aged 0–59 months who are below minus two standard deviations from median weight-for-height of the WHO Child Growth Standards.

Underweight – Moderate and severe: Percentage of children aged 0–59 months who are below minus two standard deviations from median weight-for-age of the WHO Child Growth Standards.

Overweight – Moderate and severe: Percentage of children aged 0-59 months who are above two standard deviations from median weight-for-height of the WHO Child Growth Standards.

MAIN DATA SOURCES

Under-five mortality rate – United Nations Inter-agency Group for Child Mortality Estimation (IGME). UNICEF/WHO/World Bank/United Nations Population Division, 2012.

Under-five population – United Nations Population Division.

Low birthweight – Demographic and Health Surveys (DHS), Multiple Indicator Cluster Surveys (MICS), other national household surveys, data from routine reporting systems and UNICEF.

Stunting, wasting, underweight and overweight – DHS, MICS, other national household surveys, WHO and UNICEF.

NOTES

* Data refer to the most recent year available during the period specified in the column heading.

– Data not available.

x Data refer to years or periods other than those specified in the column heading. Such data are not included in the calculation of regional and global averages, with the exception of 2005–2006 data from India.

y Data differ from the standard definition or refer to only part of a country. If they fall within the noted reference period, such data are included in the calculation of regional and global averages.

θ Regional averages for underweight (moderate and severe), stunting (moderate and severe), wasting (moderate and severe) and overweight (moderate and severe) are estimated using statistical modeling of data from the UNICEF and WHO Joint Global Nutrition Database, 2011 revision (completed July 2012).

Table 3. Infant and young child feeding practices and micronutrient indicators

Countries and areas	Annual number of births (thousands) 2011	Early initiation of breastfeeding (%) 2007–2011*	% of children (2007–2011*) who are: Exclusively breastfed (<6 months)	Introduced to solid, semi-solid or soft foods (6–8 months)	Breastfed at age 1 (12–15 months)	Breastfed at age 2 (20–23 months)	Vitamin A supplementation full coverageᐃ (%) 2011	Households with iodized salt (%) 2007–2011*
Afghanistan	1,408	–	–	29 x	92 x	54 x	100	28 x
Albania	41	43	39	78	61	31	–	76 y
Algeria	712	50 x	7 x	39 x,y	47 x	22 x	–	61 x
Andorra	–	–	–	–	–	–	–	–
Angola	803	55	11 x	77 x	89 x	37 x	55	45
Antigua and Barbuda	–	–	–	–	–	–	–	–
Argentina	693	–	–	–	55	28	–	–
Armenia	47	36	35	48 y	44	23	–	97 x
Australia	307	–	–	–	–	–	–	–
Austria	74	–	–	–	–	–	–	–
Azerbaijan	184	32 x	12 x	83 x	35 x	16 x	–	54 x
Bahamas	5	–	–	–	–	–	–	–
Bahrain	23	–	–	–	–	–	–	–
Bangladesh	3,016	36 x	64	71	95	90	94	84 x
Barbados	3	–	–	–	–	–	–	–
Belarus	107	21 x	9 x	38 x	18 x	4 x	–	94 y
Belgium	123	–	–	–	–	–	–	–
Belize	8	51 x	10 x	–	–	27 x	–	–
Benin	356	32	43 x	76 y	99	92	98	86
Bhutan	15	59	49	67	93	66	–	96 x
Bolivia (Plurinational State of)	264	64	60	83	85	40	21	89 y
Bosnia and Herzegovina	32	57 x	18 x	29 x	26 x	10 x	–	62 x
Botswana	47	40	20	46 y	36	6	75	65
Brazil	2,996	43 x	41 y	70 x	50 x	25 x	–	96 x
Brunei Darussalam	8	–	–	–	–	–	–	–
Bulgaria	75	–	–	–	–	–	–	100 x
Burkina Faso	730	20 x	25	61	97	80	87	34 x
Burundi	288	–	69	70 y	94	79	83	98 x
Cambodia	317	65	74	82 y	83	43	92	83 y
Cameroon	716	20 x	20	63 x,y	79 x	24	–	49 x
Canada	388	–	–	–	–	–	–	–
Cape Verde	10	73 x	60 x	80 x	77 x	13 x	–	75
Central African Republic	156	43	34	56 x,y	86 x	32	0	65
Chad	511	29	3	46	88	59	–	54
Chile	245	–	–	–	–	–	–	–
China	16,364	41	28	43 y	37	–	–	97 y
Colombia	910	57	43	86	59	33	–	–
Comoros	28	25 x	21 x	34 x	65 x	45 x	–	82 x
Congo	145	39 x	19 x	78 x	82 x	21 x	–	82 x
Cook Islands	–	–	–	–	–	–	–	–
Costa Rica	73	–	15 x	92	67	40	–	–
Côte d'Ivoire	679	25 x	4 x	51 x	87 x	37 x	100	84 x
Croatia	43	–	–	–	–	–	–	–
Cuba	110	70 x	49	77	25	17	–	88 x
Cyprus	13	–	–	–	–	–	–	–
Czech Republic	116	–	–	–	–	–	–	–
Democratic People's Republic of Korea	348	18	65 x	31 x	86	36	100	25 y
Democratic Republic of the Congo	2,912	43	37	52	87	53	98	59
Denmark	64	–	–	–	–	–	–	–
Djibouti	26	67	1 x	35 x	54 x	18 x	95	0 x
Dominica	–	–	–	–	–	–	–	–
Dominican Republic	216	65	8	88	34	12	–	19 x
Ecuador	298	–	40 x	77 x	62 x	23 x	–	–
Egypt	1,886	56	53	70	78	35	–	79
El Salvador	126	33	31	72 y	73	54	–	62 x
Equatorial Guinea	26	–	24 x	–	–	–	–	33 x
Eritrea	193	78 x	52 x	43 x	92 x	62 x	46	68 x
Estonia	16	–	–	–	–	–	–	–
Ethiopia	2,613	52	52	55 x	96	82	71	15 y
Fiji	18	57 x	40 x	–	–	–	–	–
Finland	61	–	–	–	–	–	–	–
France	792	–	–	–	–	–	–	–
Gabon	42	71 x	6 x	62 x	43 x	9 x	–	36 x
Gambia	67	52	34	34	94	31	93	21

Table 3. Infant and young child feeding practices and micronutrient indicators ▶

Countries and areas	Annual number of births (thousands) 2011	Early initiation of breastfeeding (%) 2007–2011*	% of children (2007–2011*) who are:				Vitamin A supplementation full coverage△ (%) 2011	Households with iodized salt (%) 2007–2011*
			Exclusively breastfed (<6 months)	Introduced to solid, semi-solid or soft foods (6–8 months)	Breastfed at age 1 (12–15 months)	Breastfed at age 2 (20–23 months)		
Georgia	51	69	55	43 y	37	17	–	100
Germany	699	–	–	–	–	–	–	–
Ghana	776	52	63	76	95	44	–	32 x
Greece	117	–	–	–	–	–	–	–
Grenada	2	–	–	–	–	–	–	–
Guatemala	473	56	50	71 y	79	46	28	76
Guinea	394	40 x	48	32 y	100	–	88	41
Guinea-Bissau	59	55	38	43	97	65	100	12
Guyana	13	43 x	33	81	62	49	–	11
Haiti	266	44 x	41 x	90 x	83 x	35 x	36	3 x
Holy See	–	–	–	–	–	–	–	–
Honduras	205	79 x	30 x	84 x	72 x	48 x	–	–
Hungary	100	–	–	–	–	–	–	–
Iceland	5	–	–	–	–	–	–	–
India	27,098	41 x	46 x	56 x	88 x	77 x	66	71
Indonesia	4,331	29	32	85	80	50	76	62 y
Iran (Islamic Republic of)	1,255	56 x	23 x	68 x	90 x	58 x	–	99 x
Iraq	1,144	31	25 x	62 x	68 x	36 x	–	28 x
Ireland	72	–	–	–	–	–	–	–
Israel	156	–	–	–	–	–	–	–
Italy	557	–	–	–	–	–	–	–
Jamaica	50	62 x	15 x	36 x	49 x	24 x	–	–
Japan	1,073	–	–	–	–	–	–	–
Jordan	154	39	22	84 y	46	11	–	88 x
Kazakhstan	345	64 x	17 x	50 x	57 x	16 x	–	92 x
Kenya	1,560	58	32	85	86	54	–	98
Kiribati	–	–	69	–	89	82	–	–
Kuwait	50	–	–	–	–	–	–	–
Kyrgyzstan	131	65 x	32 x	60 x	68 x	26 x	–	76 x
Lao People's Democratic Republic	140	30 x	26 x	41 x	82 x	48 x	92	84 x
Latvia	24	–	–	–	–	–	–	–
Lebanon	65	–	15	35 x	38	15	–	71
Lesotho	60	53	54	68	77	35	–	84
Liberia	157	44	34 y	51 y	89	41	96	–
Libya	144	–	–	–	–	–	–	–
Liechtenstein	–	–	–	–	–	–	–	–
Lithuania	35	–	–	–	–	–	–	–
Luxembourg	6	–	–	–	–	–	–	–
Madagascar	747	72	51	86	92	61	91	53
Malawi	686	58 x	72	86	96	77	96	50 x
Malaysia	579	–	–	–	–	–	–	18
Maldives	5	64	48	91	77	68	–	44 x
Mali	728	46 x	38 x	25 x	94 x	56 x	96	79 x
Malta	4	–	–	–	–	–	–	–
Marshall Islands	–	73	31	77 y	64	53	–	–
Mauritania	118	81	46	61 y	90	47 y	100	23
Mauritius	16	–	21 x	–	–	–	–	–
Mexico	2,195	18	19	27	–	–	–	91 x
Micronesia (Federated States of)	3	–	–	–	–	–	–	–
Monaco	–	–	–	–	–	–	–	–
Mongolia	65	71	59	78	82	66	85	70
Montenegro	8	25 x	19 x	35 x	25 x	13 x	–	71 x
Morocco	620	52 x	31 x	66 x	57 x	15 x	–	21 x
Mozambique	889	63	41	86	91	52	100	25
Myanmar	824	76	24	81 y	91	65	96	93
Namibia	60	71	24 x	91 x	69 x	28 x	–	63 x
Nauru	–	76	67	65 y	68	65	–	–
Nepal	722	45	70	66	93	93	91	80
Netherlands	181	–	–	–	–	–	–	–
New Zealand	64	–	–	–	–	–	–	–
Nicaragua	138	54	31	76 y	68	43	2	97 x
Niger	777	42	27	65 y	95	–	95	32
Nigeria	6,458	38	13	76	85	32	73	52
Niue	–	–	–	–	–	–	–	–

Countries and areas	Annual number of births (thousands) 2011	Early initiation of breastfeeding (%) 2007–2011*	% of children (2007–2011*) who are:				Vitamin A supplementation full coverage△ (%) 2011	Households with iodized salt (%) 2007–2011*
			Exclusively breastfed (<6 months)	Introduced to solid, semi-solid or soft foods (6–8 months)	Breastfed at age 1 (12–15 months)	Breastfed at age 2 (20–23 months)		
Norway	61	–	–	–	–	–	–	–
Oman	50	85 x	–	91 x	95 x	73 x	–	69 x
Pakistan	4,764	29	37	36 y	79	55	90	69
Palau	–	–	–	–	–	–	–	–
Panama	70	–	–	–	–	–	–	–
Papua New Guinea	208	–	56 x	76 x,y	89 x	72 x	12	92 x
Paraguay	158	47	24	67 y	38	14	–	93
Peru	591	51	71	82	77 y	55 y	–	91
Philippines	2,358	54	34	90	58	34	91	45 x
Poland	410	–	–	–	–	–	–	–
Portugal	97	–	–	–	–	–	–	–
Qatar	21	–	–	–	–	–	–	–
Republic of Korea	479	–	–	–	–	–	–	–
Republic of Moldova	44	65 x	46 x	18 x	41 x	2 x	–	60 x
Romania	221	–	16 x	41 x	–	–	–	74 x
Russian Federation	1,689	–	–	–	–	–	–	35 x
Rwanda	449	71	85	79	95	84	76	99
Saint Kitts and Nevis	–	–	–	–	–	–	–	100 x
Saint Lucia	3	–	–	–	–	–	–	–
Saint Vincent and the Grenadines	2	–	–	–	–	–	–	–
Samoa	4	88	51	71 y	72	74	–	–
San Marino	–	–	–	–	–	–	–	–
Sao Tome and Principe	5	45	51	74	92	20	44	86
Saudi Arabia	605	–	–	–	–	–	–	–
Senegal	471	23 x	39	61 x	97	51	–	47
Serbia	110	8	14	84	18	15	–	32
Seychelles	–	–	–	–	–	–	–	–
Sierra Leone	227	45	32	25	84	48	99	63
Singapore	47	–	–	–	–	–	–	–
Slovakia	58	–	–	–	–	–	–	–
Slovenia	20	–	–	–	–	–	–	–
Solomon Islands	17	75	74	81 y	84	67	–	–
Somalia	416	26 x	9 x	16 x	50 x	35 x	12	1 x
South Africa	1,052	61 x	8 x	49 x	66 x	31 x	44	–
South Sudanδ	–	–	45	21	82	38	–	54
Spain	499	–	–	–	–	–	–	–
Sri Lanka	373	80	76	87 y	92	84	–	92 y
State of Palestine	137	–	27 x	–	–	–	–	86 x
Sudanδ	–	–	41	51	88	40	–	10
Suriname	10	34 x	2 x	58 x	39 x	15 x	–	–
Swaziland	35	55	44	66	60	11	41	52
Sweden	113	–	–	–	–	–	–	–
Switzerland	77	–	–	–	–	–	–	–
Syrian Arab Republic	466	46	43	–	56	25	–	79 x
Tajikistan	194	57 y	25 x	15 x	75 x	34 x	99	62
Thailand	824	50 x	15	–	–	–	–	47 x
The former Yugoslav Republic of Macedonia	22	21	23	41	34	13	–	94 x
Timor-Leste	44	82	52	82	71	33	59	60
Togo	195	46	62	44	93	64	22	32
Tonga	3	–	–	–	–	–	–	–
Trinidad and Tobago	20	41 x	13 x	83 x	34 x	22 x	–	28 x
Tunisia	179	87 x	6 x	61 x,y	48 x	15 x	–	97 x
Turkey	1,289	39	42	68 y	67	22	–	69
Turkmenistan	109	60 x	11 x	54 x	72 x	37 x	–	87 x
Tuvalu	–	15	35	40 y	54	51	–	–
Uganda	1,545	42 x	62	75 x	87	46	60	96 x
Ukraine	494	41	18	86	26	6	–	18 x
United Arab Emirates	94	–	–	–	–	–	–	–
United Kingdom	761	–	–	–	–	–	–	–
United Republic of Tanzania	1,913	49	50	92	94	51	97	59
United States	4,322	–	–	–	–	–	–	–
Uruguay	49	59	65	35 y	45	27	–	–
Uzbekistan	589	67 x	26 x	47 x	78 x	38 x	95	53 x
Vanuatu	7	72	40	68	79	32	–	23

Table 3. Infant and young child feeding practices and micronutrient indicators

Countries and areas	Annual number of births (thousands) 2011	Early initiation of breastfeeding (%) 2007–2011*	% of children (2007–2011*) who are: Exclusively breastfed (<6 months)	Introduced to solid, semi-solid or soft foods (6–8 months)	Breastfed at age 1 (12–15 months)	Breastfed at age 2 (20–23 months)	Vitamin A supplementation full coverageΔ (%) 2011	Households with iodized salt (%) 2007–2011*
Venezuela (Bolivarian Republic of)	598	–	–	–	–	–	–	–
Viet Nam	1,458	40	17	50	74	19	99 w	45
Yemen	940	30 x	12 x	76 x	–	–	9	30 x
Zambia	622	57	61	94	94	42	72	77 x
Zimbabwe	377	69 x	31	86	87	20	56	94 y
Memorandum								
Sudan and South Sudanδ	1,447	–	–	–	–	–	–	–
SUMMARY INDICATORS#								
Sub-Saharan Africa	32,584	48	37	71	90	50	78	49
Eastern and Southern Africa	14,399	56	52	84	91	59	72	50
West and Central Africa	16,712	41	25	65	89	43	83	52
Middle East and North Africa	10,017	–	–	–	–	–	–	–
South Asia	37,402	39	47	55	87	75	73	71
East Asia and the Pacific	28,448	41	28	57	51	42 **	85 **	87
Latin America and the Caribbean	10,790	–	37	–	–	–	–	–
CEE/CIS	5,823	–	–	–	–	–	–	–
Least developed countries	28,334	52	49	68	92	64	82	50
World	135,056	42	39	60	76	58 **	75 **	75

\# For a complete list of countries and areas in the regions and subregions, see page 124.

δ Due to the cession in July 2011 of the Republic of South Sudan by the Republic of the Sudan, and its subsequent admission to the United Nations on 14 July 2011, disaggregated data for Sudan and South Sudan as separate States are not yet available for all indicators. In these cases, aggregated data are presented for Sudan pre-cession (see Memorandum item).

DEFINITIONS OF THE INDICATORS

Early initiation of breastfeeding – Percentage of infants who are put to the breast within one hour of birth.

Exclusive breastfeeding (<6 months) – Percentage of children aged 0–5 months who were fed exclusively with breastmilk during the past 24 hours.

Introduction of solid, semi-solid or soft foods (6–8 months) – Percentage of children aged 6–8 months who received solid, semi-solid or soft foods during the past 24 hours.

Continued breastfeeding at age 1 (12–15 months) – Percentage of children aged 12–15 months who received breastmilk during the past 24 hours.

Continued breastfeeding at age 2 (20–23 months) – Percentage of children aged 20–23 months who received breastmilk during the past 24 hours.

Vitamin A supplementation (full coverage) – The estimated percentage of children aged 6–59 months reached with two doses of vitamin A supplementation.

Households with iodized salt – Percentage of households consuming adequately iodized salt (15 parts per million or more).

MAIN DATA SOURCES

Annual births – United Nations Population Division.

Breastfeeding – Demographic and Health Surveys (DHS), Multiple Indicator Cluster Surveys (MICS), other national household surveys and UNICEF.

Vitamin A supplementation – UNICEF.

Households with iodized salt – DHS, MICS, other national household surveys and UNICEF.

NOTES

* Data refer to the most recent year available during the period specified in the column heading.

– Data not available.

x Data refer to years or periods other than those specified in the column heading. Such data are not included in the calculation of regional and global averages, with the exception of 2005–2006 data from India.

y Data differ from the standard definition or refer to only part of a country. If they fall within the noted reference period, such data are included in the calculation of regional and global averages.

w Identifies countries with national vitamin A supplementation programmes targeted towards a reduced age range. Coverage figure is reported as targeted.

Δ Full coverage with vitamin A supplements is reported as the lower percentage of 2 annual coverage points (i.e., lower point between round 1 [January–June] and round 2 [July–December] of 2011).

** Excludes China.

Regional classification

Sub-Saharan Africa

Eastern and Southern Africa; West and Central Africa; Djibouti; Sudan[1]

Eastern and Southern Africa

Angola; Botswana; Burundi; Comoros; Eritrea; Ethiopia; Kenya; Lesotho; Madagascar; Malawi; Mauritius; Mozambique; Namibia; Rwanda; Seychelles; Somalia; South Africa; South Sudan;[1] Swaziland; Uganda; United Republic of Tanzania; Zambia; Zimbabwe

West and Central Africa

Benin; Burkina Faso; Cameroon; Cape Verde; Central African Republic; Chad; Congo; Côte d'Ivoire; Democratic Republic of the Congo; Equatorial Guinea; Gabon; Gambia; Ghana; Guinea; Guinea-Bissau; Liberia; Mali; Mauritania; Niger; Nigeria; Sao Tome and Principe; Senegal; Sierra Leone; Togo

Middle East and North Africa

Algeria; Bahrain; Djibouti; Egypt; Iran (Islamic Republic of); Iraq; Jordan; Kuwait; Lebanon; Libya; Morocco; Oman; Qatar; Saudi Arabia; State of Palestine; Sudan;[1] Syrian Arab Republic; Tunisia; United Arab Emirates; Yemen

South Asia

Afghanistan; Bangladesh; Bhutan; India; Maldives; Nepal; Pakistan; Sri Lanka

East Asia and the Pacific

Brunei Darussalam; Cambodia; China; Cook Islands; Democratic People's Republic of Korea; Fiji; Indonesia; Kiribati; Lao People's Democratic Republic; Malaysia; Marshall Islands; Micronesia (Federated States of); Mongolia; Myanmar; Nauru; Niue; Palau; Papua New Guinea; Philippines; Republic of Korea; Samoa; Singapore; Solomon Islands; Thailand; Timor-Leste; Tonga; Tuvalu; Vanuatu; Viet Nam

Latin America and the Caribbean

Antigua and Barbuda; Argentina; Bahamas; Barbados; Belize; Bolivia (Plurinational State of); Brazil; Chile; Colombia; Costa Rica; Cuba; Dominica; Dominican Republic; Ecuador; El Salvador; Grenada; Guatemala; Guyana; Haiti; Honduras; Jamaica; Mexico; Nicaragua; Panama; Paraguay; Peru; Saint Kitts and Nevis; Saint Lucia; Saint Vincent and the Grenadines; Suriname; Trinidad and Tobago; Uruguay; Venezuela (Bolivarian Republic of)

Central and Eastern Europe and the Commonwealth of Independent States (CEE/CIS)

Albania; Armenia; Azerbaijan; Belarus; Bosnia and Herzegovina; Bulgaria; Croatia; Georgia; Kazakhstan; Kyrgyzstan; Montenegro; Republic of Moldova; Romania; Russian Federation; Serbia; Tajikistan; the former Yugoslav Republic of Macedonia; Turkey; Turkmenistan; Ukraine; Uzbekistan

Least developed countries/areas

Classified as such by the United Nations High Representative for the Least Developed Countries, Landlocked Developing Countries and Small Island Developing States (UN-OHRLLS).
Afghanistan; Angola; Bangladesh; Benin; Bhutan; Burkina Faso; Burundi; Cambodia; Central African Republic; Chad; Comoros; Democratic Republic of the Congo; Djibouti; Equatorial Guinea; Eritrea; Ethiopia; Gambia; Guinea; Guinea-Bissau; Haiti; Kiribati; Lao People's Democratic Republic; Lesotho; Liberia; Madagascar; Malawi; Mali; Mauritania; Mozambique; Myanmar; Nepal; Niger; Rwanda; Samoa; Sao Tome and Principe; Senegal; Sierra Leone; Solomon Islands; Somalia; South Sudan;[1] Sudan;[1] Timor-Leste; Togo; Tuvalu; Uganda; United Republic of Tanzania; Vanuatu; Yemen; Zambia

General note on the data

The data presented in this report are derived from UNICEF global databases, which include only internationally comparable and statistically sound data. In addition, data from the responsible United Nations organization have been used wherever possible. In the absence of such internationally standardized estimates, the profiles draw on other sources, particularly data drawn from nationally representative household surveys such as Multiple Indicator Cluster Surveys (MICS) and Demographic and Health Surveys (DHS). Data presented reflect the latest available estimates as of late 2012. More detailed information on methodology and the data sources is available at <www.childinfo.org>.

Data cannot be compared across consecutive reports: Some of the data presented in this report are subject to evolving methodologies and revisions of time series data. For other indicators, comparable data are unavailable from one year to the next. It is therefore not advisable to compare data from consecutive reports.

---

[1] Due to the cession in July 2011 of the Republic of South Sudan by the Republic of the Sudan, and its subsequent admission to the United Nations on 14 July 2011, disaggregated data for the Sudan and South Sudan as separate States are not yet available for all indicators. Aggregated data presented are for the Sudan pre-cession, and these data are included in the averages for the Middle East and North Africa, and sub-Saharan Africa regions as well as the least developed countries/areas category. For the purposes of this report, South Sudan is designated as a least developed country.